SIRTFOOD DIET

The Ultimate Guide to Boost YOUR Metabolism, Burn Fat and Get Lean. Start Losing Weight RIGHT NOW by Activating Your Skinny Gene with the Revolutionary Diet Adopted by Many Celebrities.

GEENA MOORE

DISCLAIMER

This book is meant for educational and information purposes only. It is not meant to give any medical advice, diagnose, or treat any medical conditions. No medical claims are made in this book. The nutritional advice given in this book will not treat or cure medical conditions, metabolic disorders, or other illnesses. The nutritional advice is meant for healthy individuals who want to improve their appearance for cosmetic reasons and not to treat illnesses of any kind.

You should always consult your physician or other healthcare provider should you have any questions regarding a medical condition or treatment plan.

The author is not a MD or RD and cannot be held liable or responsible to any person or entity with respect to any information contained in this book. The reader/ user assumes all risks for any injury, loss or damage caused or alleged to be caused directly or indirectly by using the information contained in this book.

Table of Contents

Introduction

New diet trends emerge at regular intervals, which are tested by stars or developed by nutrition experts. One principle that persists is low carb. A new variant of this diet, the sort food diet, is now supposed to melt fat deposits even faster.

Lose Weight with the Sirtfood Diet

The name already reveals what the diet is basically based on; so-called sort foods are all those foods that stimulate the fat-burning enzyme sit-in and reduce the extra pounds.

The basis of the sort food diet is the scientific knowledge that certain plant substances stimulate the activity of the body's own sit-ins as well as fasting. Aidan Goggin's and Glen Mitten, the nutritionists and authors of the diet bestseller of the same name, are convinced that a diet based on the sit-in principle not only leads to a dream figure but also with enjoyment. As long as you combine the relevant foods in a targeted manner and outwit your metabolism in this way.

Examples of the secondary plant substances that are considered to be sit-in activators are allicin, which gives garlic its typical aroma, capsaicin, which is mainly found in chilies, or curcumin, to which turmeric owes its yellow color.

Sirtfoods not only boost fat burning effect, but they also protect the organism from cell damage, heart or cancer diseases and slow down the general aging process. Sit-ins also prevent typical cravings, support muscle building and cellular fitness and strengthen the immune system. What makes a sit-in diet so much easier: Sirtfoods are neither particularly unusual nor boring. These are everyday foods, especially fruits and vegetables. By the way, red wine and chocolate are also allowed.

The Most important Sirtfoods for losing Weight

The basis first: All foods are plant-based in the Sirtfood diet. The valuable sit-ins provide fruit and vegetables, but also spices and herbs. Typical sort foods include apples, blueberries, raspberries and citrus fruits as well as broccoli, kale, tomatoes, arugula, onions, celery, garlic, parsley, chilly, turmeric, walnuts and cashew nuts. Sit-ins are also contained in dark chocolate with 85 percent cocoa and in red wine. These foods are supplemented with proven protein sources known from the low carb diet: soy products, white meat or eggs.

Three Phases of the Sirtfood Diet

As a diet with quick results, Aidan Goggin's and Glen Mitten recommend a strict three-phase diet plan. Fasting is similar in the first three days. With a strongly reduced diet (around 1000 calories are allowed daily), the self-cleaning process of the cells is activated and the metabolism gets going. Accordingly, you can drink three green smoothies or juices and eat a sort of food meal for three days.

The second phase should push the fat-burning further and at the same time increase the energy turnover. Specifically, 1500 calories a day are then provided in the form of two sort food juices and two sort food meals. The third phase serves to stabilize the new, slimmer silhouette and should be carried out for at least another week or longer. In addition to the still indispensable sort of foods, protein sources and essential fats are increasingly allowed here.

Chapter 1 - What Are the basic Mechanisms and Advantages of Sirtfood Diet?

Low-carb is probably the best-known principle for losing weight. You can find out what constitutes a low-carb diet and how it works here.

- **Low-Carb Diet: basics**

Low-carb is a form of nutrition (diet) in which the carbohydrates are greatly reduced and the focus of the macronutrients is on protein and fat.

The intake of carbohydrates has risen sharply in recent decades. We ingest over 50 percent of the calories consumed on average via carbohydrates. If you look at the previous diet of hunters and gatherers (22 - 40 percent carbohydrates), you can see that consumption has more than doubled in some cases.

The reasons for this lie primarily in the cheap production of many carbohydrate-rich foods, which are also highly addictive due to their sugar. In addition, fats have long been considered an enemy of nutrition.

However, the focus on carbohydrates did not combat obesity but rather increased it in some cases. Diseases like type 2 diabetes are also promoted by many bad carbohydrates. The trend towards low carb as a countermovement is understandable. But what does low carb mean anyway?

- **Low-Carb Diet: Well-Known Representatives**

But low-carb is not the same as low-carb! The term low-carbohydrate diet is quite vague and that's why there is no low-carb diet.

- Atkins diet

- Keto Diet/Anabolic Diet

- Loge method

- Dukan diet

- New York diet

- South Beach Diet

- **Low-Carb Diet: Advantages**

It works: It is not for nothing that everyone is talking about low-carb as an umbrella term for many diets. Before preparation competitions, bodybuilders almost always use low-carb to accelerate weight loss and achieve optimal shape in a short time. Studies have shown that a low-carb diet provides better results in the short term than a low-fat diet.

Health: Studies have also shown that after a period of one year, people got a better grip on various inflammation values and fat metabolism disorders through low-carb.

Saturation: Low-carb keeps blood sugar levels stable and ensures that you feel fewer cravings. The satiety effect is better overall than with low-fat diets. You also avoid fatigue after eating a high-carb meal.

- **Low-Carb Diet: Disadvantages**

Hardly any energy: a low-carb diet requires a strong will and a soft spot for foods with a lot of protein. A radical renunciation of carbohydrates will often make you feel weak and drained. If you have a physically or mentally demanding job, low-carb will quickly reach its limits.

Bad mood: Due to the lack of energy, you not only lack the power for many activities but you also quickly feel irritated or annoyed. This is because carbohydrates in the body increase the level of serotonin. The happiness hormone ensures a good mood.

Just think in the short term: Studies have shown that you can lose weight quickly with low carb. In the long run, however, the body adapts, and you won't do better compared to other diets.

Food: Every diet has its rules and with low carb, carbohydrates are largely taboo. This not only means that sugar, bread and some vegetables no longer appear on the plate, you should also avoid most fruit from now on. So, you need good low-carb recipes and a list of foods that have been deleted from now on. You can find out how to create a nutritional plan here.

- **Low-Carb Diet: 6 practical Tips**
1. Extreme low-carb diets should only be used for a short time, for example, to have a great shape on a certain day (competition, photoshoot, etc.).
2. Choose your few carbohydrates very carefully and avoid sugar. Rely on whole grains or carbohydrates with lots of fiber.
3. Low-carb alone is not successful if you do not adhere to the basic rule of weight loss: keep to a calorie deficit. So, you're eating plan should be tailored to your calories.
4. Make sure you have a healthy balance between animal and vegetable protein.

5. Be careful with special low-carb foods such as "protein bread" or "protein chips." These often contain more calories because the reduction in carbohydrates is compensated for by an increase in fat.

6. Make sure you have a balanced diet by constantly using new recipes and not eating chicken and skimmed cheese every day. This is important so that you can stick to the low-carb diet permanently and your body receives many important micronutrients.

History of Sirtfood Diet and main Contributors

Specialists found that the best wellsprings of Sirtfoods were found in the weight control plans of those bragging the most reduced rates sickness and heftiness on the planet—from the Kuna American Indians, who seem resistant to hypertension and show strikingly low paces of stoutness, diabetes, malignancy, and early passing, because of a phenomenally rich admission of the Sirtfood cocoa; to Okinawa, Japan, where a smorgasbord of Sirtfoods, smooth figures, and long life all go connected at the hip; to India, where the unquenchable craving for everything fiery, particularly the Sirtfood turmeric, has left disease afterward. In any case, the eating routine is the jealousy of the remainder of the Western world, a conventional Mediterranean eating routine, where the benefits of Sirtfoods genuinely stick out. Here heftiness doesn't win and interminable ailment is the special case, not the standard. Additional virgin olive oil, wild verdant greens, nuts, berries, red wine, dates, and herbs are for the most part intense Sirtfoods, and all components noticeably in the local Mediterranean eating routine. The scientific world has been left in amazement considering the latest accord that following a Mediterranean eating regimen is more successful than checking calories for weight reduction, and more compelling than pharmaceutical medications for halting infection.

This prompts "Predimed," a game-changing investigation of the Mediterranean eating routine, distributed in 2013. It was directed on very nearly 7,400 people at high danger of cardiovascular illness, and the outcomes were acceptable to the point that the preliminary was halted ahead of schedule—after only five years. The reason of "Predimed" was delightfully straightforward. It asked what the distinction would be between a Mediterranean-style diet enhanced with either additional virgin olive oil or nuts (particularly pecans) and a progressively traditional advanced eating routine. What's more, what a distinction it was.

The adjustment in the eating routine decreased the occurrence of cardiovascular ailment by around 30 percent, an outcome medicates organizations can just dream of. Upon further development, it was discovered that there was additionally a 30 percent fall in diabetes, alongside noteworthy drops in irritation, upgrades in memory and mind wellbeing, and a huge 40 percent decrease in weight, with remarkable fat misfortune, particularly around the stomach region.

However, at first, specialists couldn't clarify what created these emotional benefits. Neither the measures of calories, fats, and sugars are eaten—the run of the mill estimates used to survey the food we eat nor physical action levels contrasted between the gatherings to clarify the findings. There must be something different going on.

At that point, the aha second struck. Both additional virgin olive oil and pecans stand apart for their remarkable substance of sirtuin-actuating polyphenols. Basically, by adding these in noteworthy adds up to a typical Mediterranean eating regimen, what the scientists had accidentally made was a superrich Sirtfood diet, and they found that it conveyed amazing outcomes.

So scientists investigating "Predimed" concocted a smart theory. If it is the polyphenols that at last issue, they pondered, at that point the individuals who ate a large portion of them would encounter their combined benefits by living the longest. So they ran the details, and the outcomes were faltering. Over just five years, the individuals who expended the most elevated levels of polyphenols had 37 percent fewer passings contrasted with the individuals who ate the least.10 Intriguingly, this is twofold the decrease in mortality that treatment with the most regularly recommended blockbuster statin drugs is found to bring. At last, we had the clarification for the awesome benefits this investigation watched, and it was more remarkable than any medication in presence.

The analysts likewise noted something different of significance. While numerous investigations have recently discovered that individual Sirtfoods give great wellbeing benefits, they were never significant enough to expand life. "Predimed" was the first of its sort. The thing that matters was that it took a gander at an example of nourishments as opposed to a solitary food. Various nourishments give distinctive sirtuin-enacting polyphenols, which work in amicability to create a significantly more impressive result than any single food can. This left us with an unstoppable end. Genuine wellbeing isn't procured through one single supplement or even one "wonder food." What you need is an entire eating regimen filled with a mix of Sirtfoods all working in collaboration. Furthermore, this is the thing that prompted the production of the Sirtfood Diet.

Chapter 2 - Theory and how It Works on Metabolism

Now, this all may sound too good to be true at this point in time. How is it potentially possible that you can do all of that just with the use of the Sirtfood diet? How can you ever hope to change the way in which your body will respond to the calorie restrictions? If most of the time, fasting and calorie restriction impact the metabolism, how is it that sirtfoods would not? These are all very important questions to keep in mind, and if you are looking at doing something to your body, such as restricting calories, you are absolutely in the right, asking questions about how what you are doing will work and impact your body. Rest assured—your questions will be answered. Here, we are going to answer four key questions. What are sirtuins? How do sirtuins work for the body? How does calorie restriction impact the body? What are the effects of eating Sirtuins-rich foods? As you read, hopefully, you will get an idea of what it is that you can come to expect if you decide that this is the diet for you.

What Are Sirtuins?

Sirtuins is the name for a whole host of proteins that are there to regulate the health of your cells. They help your body to maintain cellular homeostasis, which is a fancy way of saying that they keep the cells balanced to the specifications that they are supposed to be. Homeostasis is found when your body has functions that keep it in the same condition constantly, which is why your body is usually always at right around 98.6 degrees Fahrenheit—that is a way that your body maintains homeostasis. Likewise, your cells have a process to keep them in homeostasis as well—the sirtuins.

Proteins in your body are the workers, essentially, they work to serve very specific roles to keep your body functioning. Think of your body as one big corporation. Within your body, you have different sorts of parts; there are the organs, which serve sort of like the management of a corporation. You have nerves, which connect everything together like a network of computers. You have proteins—these are like individual departments within your particular corporation. Think about it—a corporation will have customer service, human resources, and all sorts of other departments within it so that it can function properly. They are all departments—but they are each responsible for a different role. Proteins in the body are similar; they are like the departments that keep everything going. When you take a look at sirtuins, you are looking at a department of proteins that is capable of providing your cells with a way that it can keep the body functioning. In terms of the Sirtfood Diet, they are recognized as the parts that can activate the "skinny gene"—they tell your body to let go of the fats.

How Do Sirtuins Work?

You have seven sirtuins in your body—three of them are designed to work in the mitochondria, three of them work in the nucleus, where your DNA is stored so that cells can be run and regulated, and one more is kept in the cytoplasm. They all work together and have very different roles, but they all do one thing: remove acetyl groups from proteins.

Acetyl groups are able to alter and control the reactions that a cell has—they are like barcodes on proteins that tell other proteins what they are and how to interact with them. Through the process of deacetylation, sirtuins work to recognize that a molecule in the body has an acetyl group and they then move it, allowing the molecule to get ready to do its job. Essentially, the sirtuins are able to get everything ready to work.

In terms of the Sirtfood Diet, then you can expect that the act of fasting and restricting calories will change the way that the body is working. It will then allow for the sirtuins throughout the body to have an effect on how it works. Fat synthesis is repressed. The body is told not to uptake the cholesterol. The body is able to reject the fatty acids. Because fasting will up the level of activation of sirtuins, it allows for fats to not be stored. They are activated for use instead, allowing the body to burn them for energy when it is needed. The barcodes for those acetyl groups on the fats in the body essentially get scanned, and the sirtuins tell the molecule to get ready for work—which in this case, will be making use of the way that the body processes it. The fat goes through oxidation, gets used up, and therefore is lost from the body.

The Role of Sirtuins in Aging and Age-Related Diseases

The first sirtuin, called SIR2, was discovered by Dr. Amar Klar in the 1970s as a gene that controls the capacity of leaven cells to mate. Years later, in the 1990s, researchers identified specific genes that were — identical in form — homologous to SIR2 in certain species such as mice, fruit flies, also called sirtuins. Each organism had different numbers of sirtuins. For starters, yeast has five sirtuins, one has bacteria, seven have mice, and seven have humans.

In 1991, along with Nick Austriaco and Brian Kennedy, Elysium's co-founder and MIT scientist Leonard Guarente performed research on how yeast was aging. Luckily, Austriaco tried to grow yeast crops from samples that he had been storing for months in his fridge that produced a stressful environment for the strains. Many of the strains could only develop from here, but Guarente and his team established a pattern: the yeast strains which lasted the best in the refrigerator were also the most extended living. This led Guarente to focus solely on these long-lived strains of yeast.

This contributed to SIR2 being identified as a gene that facilitated yeast survival. It is important to note that there is no evidence to date that this study can be extrapolated to humans, and further research on the effects of SIR2 on humans is necessary. The Guarente lab, therefore, observed that eliminating SIR2 shortened leaven life significantly, although growing the number of copies of the SIR2 gene from one to two, increased the yeast life period. Yet, of course, what triggered SIR2 has yet to be identified.

This is where groups of acetyl come into play. At first, it was believed that SIR2 could be an enzyme deacetylating — which indicates that certain acetyl groups were separated — from other molecules. Still, no one understood if that was valid, as all attempts to demonstrate that behavior in a test tube proved negatively. Guarente and his colleagues observed that in the presence of NAD+, nicotinamide adenine dinucleotide, SIR2 in yeast could only deacetylate specific proteins.

Benefits of Keto Diet vs. Benefits of Sirtfood Diet

Let's realize it. How does the human body really find that many various forms of slimming down?

Every year there appears to be some revolutionary diet rolling in hot off the press with the encouragement of several big celebrities. It makes its major debut, and thanks to the front of every famous magazine in the checkout line of the grocery store. Another fitness advocate who featured on a well-known chat show discussing the facts behind this modern form of dieting, as though it were a brand different discovery.

Still, you can't help but wonder if perhaps this one is going to be the trick So the days of doing whatever you like the hell you can without receiving a single pound are done, at least until maturity says sorry love. There have been two eating programs over the past few years which have been fighting it out in the spotlight. There's a low-carb, high-fat Keto diet and a "skinny gene" diet that boosts Sirtfood.

Keep tight. What divides the two? Which are the better targets for your health and weight loss? What constitutes a "skinny gene" in the world?! Let's discover everything there's to learn about every diet to address your questions.

What is the Diet of Keto?

Let's start with the keto diet or ketogenic diet. In brief, a keto diet consists of minimal carbohydrate consumption, balanced fats, and high-fat products. True keto peeps strive to eat 20 g or less of carbohydrates, a day-consuming most of their calories from healthy fat.

Invented by Peter Hutten ocher back in the 1970s, the theory behind this is that the body can reach a "ketosis" condition. What is it that now? It is yet another sophisticated way of suggesting that the body ceases depending on glycogen and starts to eat carbon instead. Essentially, as you reduce your consumption of carb and calories, your body (especially your liver) creates tiny molecules called ketones that function while your blood sugar levels are small, to supply your body with energy.

Ketones are made from fat, so your body is reprogrammed to run on fat, as opposed to glucose on this diet. By restricting your calorie consumption and, in a sense, teaching your body to use fat for food, it can then start accessing fat reserves in your body as it requires energy. It seems reasonable, right?

Advantages of the Keto Diet vs. Sirtfood Diet

Both of these common diets tend to encourage you to consume a broad range of foods that many diets enable you to cut out to meet your objectives for weight loss. They deliver a menu that is far more practical and enjoyable than the cabbage soup diet, let us claim. Now the main problem is: which one is best for your safety and for you?

The keto diet will help you shed weight, and it also has other health benefits. This will also cover up wrinkles, boost heart and brain function, and decrease the chance of life-threatening illnesses and other cancers. This has also been said to help in minimizing the epilepsy of small children.

Studies have proven that you can adhere to a mostly ketogenic food program for the long term, but adding more carbs into your diets, such as potatoes, fruits, and beans, is vital to your optimal wellbeing. On the other side, it has also been vouched for adopting a Sirtfood diet as a way to accomplish fast weight loss. This will defend you from chronic illnesses, plus it has anti-aging capabilities. Whether or not you are stringent with this diet schedule, adding these nutrient-rich Sirtfood into your diet will help your wellbeing.

But for a variety of reasons, this lifestyle is not practical in the long run. The ultra-low calorie and low carb diet may be dangerous, and much-needed work needs to be conducted to establish the effects it has on our bodies.

The bottom line is that the keto and Sirtfood diets concentrating on consuming nutrient-rich products and triggering a healthy response in our bodies resulting in higher digestion, decreased inflammation, and increased fat burning. And both diets are pretty similar.

Chapter 3 - What Is Sirtfood?

This Diet relies on research sirtuins (SIRTs), a set of seven proteins utilized from the human anatomy that's been proven to modulate various purposes, including inflammation, metabolism, and life span. Certain Natural plant chemicals could possibly find a way to grow the degree of those proteins inside the human anatomy, and foods containing them are known "sirtfoods."

The Diet blends sirtfoods and calorie limitation, both of which may possibly cause the human body to generate high degrees of sirtuins. The Sirtfood Diet publication comprises meal plans and recipes to follow along; however, there are lots of additional Sirtfood Diet recipe books out there.

The Diet's founders claim that after a Sirtfood Diet can cause accelerated body weight loss while maintaining muscles and protecting you in chronic illness. Once you've finished the dietary plan, you're invited to keep on adding sirtfoods and also the diet signature green juice to your normal diet.

Thus much, there aren't any persuasive signs that the Sirtfood Diet features a more favorable impact on weight loss than every other calorie-restricted diet regime. Along with although a number of those foods have healthy properties, there have yet to be any long-term human studies to ascertain if eating a diet full of sirtfoods has some concrete health benefits.

Nonetheless, the Sirtfood Diet publication reports the outcomes of a pilot study conducted with both the writers and between 3 9 participants in their exercise center. Nevertheless, the consequences of the study appear never to have already been released somewhere else.

To get 1 week, the participants followed the diet and worked out each day. At the close of the week, the participants lost an average of 5 pounds (3.2 kg) and claimed even gained muscle tissue. Yet these outcomes are hardly surprising. Restricting your own calorie intake to 1000 calories and exercising at the exact same period will almost always trigger weight loss.

No matter This type of fast fat reduction is neither true nor long-term, which analysis failed to accompany participants following the initial week to determine whether they attained some of the weight, and this is an average of the situation. When your own body is energy-deprived, it melts away its catastrophe energy stores, or glycogen, along with burning off muscle and fat.

Each Molecule of glycogen necessitates 3-4 atoms of water to bestow. Whenever your body melts away glycogen, then it eliminates the water too. It's referred to as "water." The very first week of extreme calorie limit, just about one-fifth of those fat loss arises from fat, whereas one other two-thirds stems out of water, glycogen, and muscle.

When your calories grow, the own body accomplishes its own glycogen stores, and also, the weight comes back again. Regrettably, such a calorie restriction may also cause the human body to reduce its metabolism, which makes it need fewer calories every day for energy compared to previously.

Additionally, it is very likely that diet might help you drop a couple of pounds at the start, although it is going to probably return once the diet has ended. As Much as preventing illness, three weeks might be long enough to own some measurable long-term effects. The flip side, adding sirtfoods to a routine diet within the long-term, might just be a fantastic idea. However, in this circumstance, you may too, bypass the diet and begin doing this today.

Top Twenty Sirtfoods

Arugula

Arugula (also known as a missile, rucola, rugula, and roquette). A pungent green salad leaf with a distinctive peppery flavor soon ascended from humble beginnings as the base of many Mediterranean peasant dishes to becoming an emblem of food snobbery in the United States.

Buckwheat

Buckwheat was one of Japan's first domesticated grains, and the legend goes that when Buddhist Buckwheat is so good that this was all they wanted, and it kept them up for weeks.

Capers

The caper bush's flower buds that grow abundantly in the Mediterranean before being picked and preserved by hand. Studies now show that capers possess essential antimicrobial, ant diabetic, anti-inflammatory, immunomodulatory, and antiviral properties, and have a long tradition of being used as a medicine in the Mediterranean and North Africa.

Celery

Celery was commonly considered a medicinal plant, particularly for washing and detoxification to prevent disease. This is especially interesting considering that the protection of liver, kidneys, and intestines is one of the many positive benefits.

Chilies

Chili has been an important part of gastronomic history worldwide for thousands of years. Its pungent fire, caused by a substance called capsaicin in chilies, is developed as a mechanism of plant defense to inflict pain and dissuade predators from feasting on it, and we appreciate that.

Cocoa

Cocoa has amazing health benefits. It's no surprise to hear that cocoa was considered a holy food for ancient cultures like the Aztecs and Mayans, and was typically reserved for the powerful and the soldiers, consumed at feasts to win allegiance and service.

Coffee

Coffee is a healthy food that is bona fide. Indeed, it is a real treasure chest of fantastic nutrients that trigger sirtuin. Becoming America's number one source of polyphenols.

Extra Virgin Olive Oil

Olive oil is the most popular of Mediterranean traditional diets. The olive tree is among the world's oldest-known planted plants, also known as the "immortal tree." And after people began pressing olives in stone mortars to harvest them, the oil has been worshipped, almost 7,000 years ago. Hippocrates cited it as a cure-all; today, a few decades later, scientific medicine confidently claims the wonderful health effects.

Garlic

Garlic has been considered one of Nature's miracle foods for thousands of years, with soothing and rejuvenating properties. Garlic is a potent natural antibiotic and antifungal that is sometimes used to help cure ulcers in the stomach.

Matcha (Green Tea)

Green tea, the toast of the Orient, and ever more common in the West. With the increasing awareness of its health benefits, green tea intake is related to less cancer, heart disease, diabetes, and osteoporosis. It is believed that green tea is so healthy for us that it is largely due to its rich content of a group of strong plant compounds called catechins, the star of the show being a special form of sirtuin-activating catechin known as epigallocatechin gallate (EGCG).

Kale

The explanation we're pro-kale is that it contains bumper numbers of the quercetin and kaempferol sirtuin-activating nutrients, rendering it a must-include in the Sirtfood Diet and the source of our green Sirtfood drink.

Medjool Dates

Medjool dates in a list of foods that encourage weight loss and promote health—especially when we tell you that Medjool dates contain a whopping 66 percent sugar. Sugar doesn't have any sirtuin-activating effects at all; instead, it has well-established connections to obesity, heart disease, and diabetes — just the reverse of what we're looking to do.

Parsley

Parsley is something of a culinary conundrum. It so often occurs in recipes, but too often, it's the green token man. At best, we serve a pair of chopped sprigs and tossed as an afterthought on a plate, at worst a single sprig for decorative purposes only. This way, there on the plate, it is always languishing even after we have stopped feeding.

Red Endive

Endive is a pretty new kid on the block in so far as vegetables go. The farmer stored chicory roots in his cellar, and then used them as a type of coffee substitute, only to forget them. Upon his return, he discovered that white leaves had sprouted, which he found to be tender, crunchy, and rather delicious upon degustation.

Red Onions

With such a long tradition of use and such strong health-giving properties, many civilizations that came before us have worshipped onions. They were held particularly by the Egyptians as objects of worship, seeing their circle-within-a-circle form as indicative of everlasting existence. And the Greeks assumed that onions made athletes better.

Red wine

The French phenomenon made headlines in the early 1990s, with it being revealed that with the French seeming to do something wrong when it came to health (smoking, lack of fitness, and rich food consumption), they had lower death rates from heart disease than countries like the United States.

Soy

Soy products have a long tradition as an important part of the diet of many countries in Asia-Pacific, such as China, Japan, and Korea. Researchers first turned on to soy after discovering that high soy-consuming countries had substantially lower rates of certain cancers, especially breast and prostate cancers.

Strawberries

Berries are powerhouses of nutrition, strawberries are earning their top twenty Sirtfood status due to their abundance of the fisetin sirtuin activator. And now studies support regular eating strawberries to promote healthy aging, staying off Alzheimer's, cancer, diabetes, heart disease, and osteoporosis.

Turmeric

Turmeric is used to treat skin disorders such as acne, psoriasis, dermatitis, and rash, along with the advantages of the "golden spice" Before Indian weddings, there is a ritual where the turmeric paste is added as a skincare treatment to the bride and groom but also to symbolize the warding off darkness.

Walnuts

Walnuts lead the way as the number one nut for health, according to the NuVal system, which ranks foods according to how nutritious they are and has been endorsed by the American College of Preventive Medicine. Yet what truly makes walnuts stand out for us is how they fly in the face of traditional thinking: they are rich in fat and calories, but well-established for weight loss and the chance of metabolic disorders like cardiovascular disease and diabetes is reduced.

Other Sirtfood

Below we listed another forty foods that we discovered have Sirtfood properties too. They strongly urge you to add these foods to sustain and promote your weight reduction and health while you further broaden your diet collection.

Vegetables

- Broccoli

- Bokchoy/pack Choi

- Asparagus

- Artichokes

- Yellow endive

- Watercress

- White onions

- Green beans

- Shallots

- Frisée

Fruits

- Red grapes

- Raspberries

- Goji berries

- Cranberries

- Black plums

- Black currants

- Kumquats

- Blackberries

- Apples

Nuts and seeds

- Sunflower seeds

- Pistachio nuts

- Pecan nuts

- Peanuts

- Chia seeds

- Chestnuts

Grains and pseudo-grains

- Whole-wheat flour

- Quinoa

- Popcorn

Beans

- White beans (e.g., cannellini or navy)

- Fava beans

Herbs and spices

- Ginger

- Dried sage

- Dried oregano

- Dill (fresh and dried)

- Cinnamon

- Chives

- Peppermint (fresh and dried)

- Thyme (fresh and dried)

Beverages

- White tea

- Black tea

Protein Power

A high protein diet is one of the most common diets in the last few years. Higher protein intake while dieting has been shown to encourage satiety, sustain metabolism, and reduce muscle mass loss. Yet it's when they pair Sirtfoods with protein that things get taken to a whole new level.

Chapter 4 - Potential Health Benefits of Sirtfood Diet

Sirtfood diet has vast health benefits. Besides weight reduction and the presence of low-calorie levels that help in the burning of fats and, consequently, weight reduction, the sirtfood diet has many health benefits, as below. These sirtfoods have higher levels of a wide range of nutrients and properties that have many health benefits.

Sirtfood Diet in Weight Reduction

Sirtfood diet helps mainly in weight loss. The diet contains much of the sirtuin proteins, which triggers the body to burn more fat for energy used in the body. Additionally, the sirtfood diet has low-calorie concentration, and this helps in less fat build-up in the body. Studies have shown that, with increased levels of sirtuins proteins in the body, there are increased levels of fat loss. With increased weight reduction in the body, a person is protected from common diseases that result from fat build-up. Some of those diseases include high blood pressure and stroke. The most effective sirtfood diets which increase sirtuin proteins in the body consist of green juice, coffee, and soy. Hence, a sirtfood diet is beneficial in enhancing weight loss.

Nutrients Absorption Enhancement

The sirtfood diet helps in easy nutrient absorption and increased energy levels in the body. The most effective sirtfood diet with these characteristics is the green juice. Nutrients from the sirtfood diet are readily available hence readily absorbed in the body. With the increased availability of nutrients is easy absorption of nutrients and, consequently, increased energy levels in the body. The kale juice, which is commonly used in the making of the green juice is very useful in enhancing nutrient absorption. These nutrients present includes vitamins, proteins, healthy fats, and water. Thus, the sirtfood diet has a health benefit of improving and enhancing nutrient absorption.

Sirtfood Diet with Brain Improvement, Skin, Hair and Nail Growth

The sirtfood diet is very useful in improving the health of the skin, enhancing healthy hair and nails, and improving the cognitive function of the brain. Commonly used sirtfood diet with this characteristic of enhancing healthy and glowing skin and strong hair and nails is kales. Additionally, cognitive function is improved by stimulation of the nervous system and the presence of minerals that enhance brain development. Sirtfood diet, which enhances cognitive function, includes coffee, kales, blueberries, and dark chocolate. Thus, a sirtfood diet is beneficial for strengthening mental health, skin development, and healthy nails and hair.

Diabetes, Tumors and Cancer Prevention

Sirtfood is very useful in the prevention of common types of illnesses such as diabetes, tumors, and cancer. Most of the sirtfood diet components contain anti-oxidants that are important in the prevention and treatment of tumors, cancer, and diabetes. Soy, capers, and extra virgin olive oil are the most effective sirtfoods used for this purpose. The development of tumors is prevented by inhibiting tumor oxidants. In addition to that, diabetes is mostly triggered by sugar levels and insulin in the body. These sirtfoods reduce and balance sugar levels in the body, thus preventing and treating the diseases. Cancer is mostly caused by inflammation of the cells, and these sirtfoods are very useful in inhibiting cell inflammation. All the sirtfoods with anti-oxidation properties can help in the prevention of cancer and tumors.

Energy Building with Sirtfood Diet

The majority of people lack enough energy in the body. With sirtfoods, their energy levels are boosted. Energy-boosting in the body is enhanced by stimulation of the brain, for example, by coffee and turmeric. The presence of proteins in the sirtfood diet assists in raising the energy levels in the body. The diet mostly has low glycemic indexes, thus their energizing properties. Water is also a significant component of the sirtfood diet, and it helps in energy-boosting. Mostly in fruits, the large percentage is water. Thus, sirtfood have the health benefit of energy-boosting in the body. Also, with fast absorption of nutrients, energy is boosted.

Enhancement of Physiological Processes and Appetite

Sirtfoods helps in improving physiological processes in the body and enhancement of appetite. Physiological processes include digestion and excretion. Common sirtfoods that will enhance metabolism and excretion include blueberries and Medjool dates. Besides that, the red chicory is a major sirtfood that increases appetite. Improved appetite is healthy and enhances the presence of nutrients in the body. Digestion is enhanced by the natural breakdown of foods and nutrients intakes in the body. Thus, sirtfoods health benefits of improving metabolism and appetite are very vital.

Sirtfood Diet with Cardiovascular Diseases

Cardiovascular diseases are prevalent types of illnesses that can be controlled by sirtfoods. This is by enhancing the health heart health and reduction of excess fats surrounding the heart that can cause heart diseases. The majority of people who consume sirtfoods reduces their probability of contracting cardiovascular diseases. Common sirtfoods that can enhance heart health and reduces risks of cardiovascular illnesses include red wine, capers, parsley, and dark chocolate. Hence, the consumption of sirtfoods is very healthy since the chances of getting heart diseases are reduced.

Treatment of Cancer, Tumors, and Use in Pain Therapy

Despite the treatment and prevention of cancer, some sirtfoods are used in cancer treatment. This is by the manufacturing of medicines that reduces pain in cancer patients. Commonly used sirtfood is lovage. Additionally, patients undergoing treatments of tumors and those with underlying urinary tract infections such as kidney stones experience much pain in their daily activities. Thus, with this sirtfoods, such patients can reduce the pain that comes as a result of such illnesses. Therefore sirtfoods have a vast range of health benefits such as the manufacturing of medicine.

Sirtfood Diet with Tissue and Muscle Development

Sirtfoods enhances muscle and tissue development. This is because it comprises all the essential nutrients in the body. Sirtfood diet provides necessary vitamins, minerals, and nutrients that keep the body and the mind very strong. Deficiencies in the body impair the body tissues and organs. Lack of essential nutrients such as vitamins, zinc, calcium phosphorous, proteins, and healthy fats leads to weak muscle and tissue development. Consequently, the risks of diseases are increased. Thus, sirtfoods are very important in proper tissue development, and this leads to a sound immune system and improving brain capacity.

Sirtfood Diet with other Types of Illnesses

Other types of health disorders that can be controlled by sirtfoods include arthritis, weak bones, and acidy in the body. Arthritis patients suffer from joint pains. These types of illnesses can be controlled by a sirtfood diet such as chilies. Blueberries are a significant source of minerals such as calcium, iron and phosphorous, and calcium. These minerals are beneficial in enhancing strong bones. Additionally, most people who have acidity problems can control this by consumption of green juice, particularly from kales. This juice is beneficial in alkalizing the body, and such patients can easily find their cure by consuming this sirtfood. Thus, sirtfood diet is very healthy in controlling such kind of illnesses.

Can the Sirtfood Diet Be good for you?

Rob notes that one positive thing about the diet is that all the foodstuffs you will consume on the menu are right for you, and your overall consumption is likely to be high. He adds, however, that any diet that cuts out entire food groups could be harmful. 'Any good study does not support the notion of flipping on the skinny gene'. The Sirtfood menu as a whole is very limited in food and calories, which can make it hard to adhere to. There is also no evidence that it is safer than any other calorie-controlled diet to lose weight. In other words, if you want to lose weight, why not eat food you would want to eat when you are mindful of the overall consumption of your calories? (And, while you are here, read our favorite fat-loss breakfast).

Who Should Avoid the Sirtfood Diet?

Rob says he's not going to support someone trying to eat with diabetes. Furthermore, he adds that it might be difficult if you are highly involved. If you go ahead, he advises that in the first part of this program, he expects side effects such as headaches or lightheadedness as the body adapts to low-calorie intake. The core concept behind the sirtfood diet is that it stimulates the mechanism of fat loss in the body and enhances muscle mass production. Nonetheless, after learning the first two phases, the question emerges: what happens after the third week of diet? Okay, the sirtfood food is for those who just enjoyed the early two stages of the diet and want to start more healthily. The diet for Sirtfood is not only just a diet for three weeks but also a way of life to follow this diet schedule. This diet is so successful and nutritious that people who have seen the effects are undoubtedly motivated to start consuming green juices every day and consume sirloin steak. Even if it is not possible to adhere to that diet every day, just having healthy food and adding a little sirtfood to it will benefit your body very much. A pilot study by Aidan and Glen, a dietary drug specialist, showed that people lose almost 7 lbs in seven days without any reduction in muscle mass. Such people have registered an improvement in strength, increased sleep, and better skin.

Despite the myriad health benefits that sirtfoods pose, there a group of people that are advised not to take sirtfoods. One group of people in this category is people with prevailing health conditions like diabetes. Medical experts argue that stringent diets like the Sirt food diet may deprive the body of essential sugars, which may worsen the status of a diabetic patient. Also, people under medication due to various body issues may have complications if they settle to the Sirt food diet. However, if the diet is complemented with other foods, the benefits are immeasurable. Apart from the few exempted individuals, sirtfoods are recommended for anyone who seeks to stay in shape.

Chapter 5 - Healthy Habits that May Increase the Efficacy of Sirtfood Diet

The basis of the sirtuin diet can be explained in simple terms or in complex ways. It is important to understand how and why it works, however, so that you can appreciate the value of what you are doing. It is important to also know why these sirtuin rich foods help to help you maintain fidelity to your diet plan. Otherwise, you may throw something in your meal with less nutrition that would defeat the purpose of planning for one rich in sirtuins. Most importantly, this is not a dietary fad, and as you will see, there is much wisdom contained in how humans have used natural foods even for medicinal purposes, over thousands of years.

To understand how the sirtfood diet works, and why these particular foods are necessary, we will look at the role they play in the human body.

Sirtuin activity was first researched in yeast, where a mutation caused an extension in the yeast's lifespan. Sirtuins were also shown to slow aging in laboratory mice, fruit flies, and nematodes. As research on sirtuins proved to transfer to mammals, they were examined for their use in diet and slowing the aging process. The sirtuins in humans are different in type, but they essentially work in the same ways and reasons.

There are seven "members" that make up the sirtuin family. It is believed that sirtuins play a big role in regulating certain functions of cells, including proliferation (reproduction and growth of cells), apoptosis (death of cells). They promote survival and resist stress to increase longevity.

They are also seen to block neurodegeneration (loss of function of the nerve cells in the brain). They conduct their housekeeping functions by cleaning out toxic proteins and supporting the brain's ability to change and adapt to different conditions, or to recuperate (i.e., brain plasticity). As part of this, they also help reduce chronic inflammation and reduce something called oxidative stress. Oxidative stress is when there are too many cell-damaging free radicals circulating in the body, and the body cannot catch up by combating them with anti-oxidants. These factors are related to age-related illness and weight as well, which again, brings us back to a discussion of how they actually work.

You will see labels in sirtuins that start with "sir," which represents "silence information regulator" genes. They do exactly that, silence or regulate, as part of their functions. The seven sirtuins that humans work with are: sirt1, sirt2, sirt3, sirt4, sirt 5, sirt6, and sirt7. Each of these types is responsible for different areas of protecting cells. They work by either stimulating or turning on certain gene expressions, or by reducing and turning off other gene expressions. This essentially means that they can influence genes to do more or less of something, most of which they are already programmed to do.

Through enzyme reactions, each of the sirt types affects different areas of cells that are responsible for the metabolic processes that help to maintain life. This is also related to what organs and functions they will affect.

After you've filled your head with more molecular biological information that you probably needed in high school or college, let's take a look at the following steps on how to follow the diet and fill your fridge. It is effortless to start the sirt food diet. It only takes a little preparation. If you don't know what kale is or where you can find green tea, you may have a learning curve, albeit a tiny one. There are a few ways to start the sirt diet.

While you prepare and cook healthy food, you may want to do a few things over the next week:

1. Clean your cupboards and refrigerator of foods that are unhealthy and might tempt you. They also have a deficient calorie intake, and you don't want to be tempted to find a quick fix that could slow you down. Even if you have new recipes, you may think your old comfort foods are now more comfortable.

2. Buy all the ingredients you need for the week. If you buy what you need, it's more profitable. Once you see the recipes, you will notice that there are many overlapping ingredients. You will know your portions when dieting, but at least you have what you need, and you will save yourself a few trips to the store.

3. Wash, dry, cut and store all the food you need so you can easily prepare it when you need it. This will make a new diet less annoying.

A necessary kitchen tool that you need in addition to real food is a juicer. You will need a juicer as soon as the sirt diet begins. Centrifuges are everywhere, so they're relatively easy to find, but the quality varies a lot. This is where price, function and comfort come in. You can go to a famous department store or find them online. Once you know what you are looking for, you can look around.

Combine Exercise with Sirtfood Diet to Be successful and Track your Diet Progress

Burns fat strengthens muscles and improves cellular physical condition: these are the guaranteed results of the Sirtfood diet. Being healthy and losing weight is a daily option. You need to take these first steps to see how it can change you and your life.

If you want to get fantastic results from Sirtfoods, here are some suggestions on how to start your diet:

Safety first

Before starting a particular food or treatment, contact your doctor, especially if you have an existing illness. This ensures that the eating does not sabotage any medications that you are taking or that are harmful to your health. Don't worry; the Sirtfood diet is pretty safe.

Knowledge Is Power

This diet is still new, but there is always the right amount of information and closer because this diet is rapidly gaining popularity. Also, you can search the Internet for recipes, food alternatives, nutrient levels and much more.

Follow the Directions

Sirtfood guarantees result if and only if you follow precisely the recommended nutritional guidelines and foods.

Help yourself

In addition to the diet program instructions, you can first remove processed and starchy foods from your healthy diet. Stop eating garbage! This will speed up the results of the SirtFood diet.

Start physical Activity

The Sirtfood diet can burn these fats and build muscle, but I recommend adding physical activity to your daily routine. Walking for 30 minutes a day would do wonders for your body and also speed up the results. Also, there are many incredible effects of training, e.g. For example: preventing and fighting health problems, improving mood, promoting better sleep, burning calories, boosting energy and much more.

Go to the Supermarket

The Sirtfood diet depends on certain foods. These foods have been selected for their ability to activate sirtuins. So if you don't follow the list, you won't see any results. Don't worry, and I will provide you with a list of recommended foods. Also, there are no overpriced foods, and you can find them almost anywhere (there may even be something hiding in your fridge).

Be prepared with the Initial "Restrictions"

If you want to obtain different results, you have to "sacrifice" a little to benefit from all the benefits of the Sirtfood diet. Don't worry, though, the first three days are the hardest for this diet as there are calorie restrictions, but rest assured that it gets easier every day. Although the restrictions imposed were not as severe for those who tried the diet, the reason was careful planning of meals. You will not be hungry with this diet if you choose wisely.

Plan your Meals

Whatever your diet, planning your meals is helpful. This not only reduces the stress of eating but also gives you the ability to weigh your selection and fill your cupboard. For the first phase of this diet, you need to do a calorie count. You will be amazed that there are many dishes with fewer calories and plenty of sirtuins.

Hire a dietary Partner

This diet can also benefit your family, your partner or your friends (not only those who are overweight). It's also more comfortable if you have a responsible partner who calls you back, shares recipes or even cooks dishes.

Document your Progress

You can start by taking "before" photos and make the required body measurements. You can also keep a food diary to track your food intake. Watch the changes in your body every week or phase. You can also have several goals to encourage him further to continue the diet.

Be careful to yourself

Don't set too many expectations. Yes, some can quickly lose 7 pounds in a week, but keep in mind that not all of our bodies are the same; and of course, your commitment counts. Other variables could be adding a workout plan to the diet plan, which could speed up the weight loss process.

Here Are some other Tips to Get you Started

Drink your juice as the first meal of the day if it helps. It's a great way to start the day for three reasons.

1. It gives you energy for breakfast and especially for lunch. By not having to digest heavy foods, your body saves the time and energy that is normally spent moving things around to perform all the tedious movements. They guarantee that you will feel lighter and more energetic that way. You can change this template at any time after the maintenance phase, but you may want to keep this schedule.

2. Having starchy foods or cooked fruits and vegetables before meals, no matter how healthy the ingredients, is the best way to digest them. Fruits and vegetables are digested faster and break down into compounds that we can use more easily. Think you have your salad before dinner. It works the same way. Heavier foods, grains, oils, meat, etc. take longer to digest. If you eat this first, they slow things down, and there you have a backup of the food that needs to be extracted. This is also the case when indigestion can occur.

3. Juices, especially greens, contain phytochemicals that not only serve as antioxidants but also contribute to our energy and mood. You will find that after drinking a green juice, you will feel very different from having eggs and sausage. You may want to keep a food journal and write things like that!

Be prepared for a lighter breakfast for a while. We often fill up on protein-rich, high-carbohydrate, and high-calorie meals early in the day. We feel that we have not eaten enough and that we are not full at first. Curiously, we can even lose chewing. Some people have to chew their food to feel like they have eaten a big meal. It's automatic that we don't think. Some will also miss this crunch, like toast. Just be careful and know that this is normal and will happen.

Chapter 6 - Main FAQ on Sirtfood Diet

Would it Be advisable for me to Exercise during Stage 1?

Ordinary exercise is perhaps the best thing you can accomplish for your wellbeing, and doing some direct exercise will improve the weight-loss and medical advantages of Stage 1 of the diet. When in doubt, we urge you to proceed with your typical degree of activity and physical movement through the initial seven days of the Sirtfood Diet. Be that as it may, we recommend remaining inside your typical safe place, since delayed or excessively exceptional exercise may basically put a lot of weight on the body for this period. Tune in to your body. There's no compelling reason to push you to accomplish more exercise during Stage 1; let the Sirtfoods accomplish the difficult work.

I'm Now thin—Would I Be Able to in any Case Follow the Diet?

We don't suggest Stage 1 of the Sirtfood Diet for any individual who is underweight. A decent method to see whether you are underweight is to compute your weight record or BMI. For whatever length of time that you know your tallness and weight, you can without much of a stretch decide this by utilizing one of the various BMI number crunchers on the web. In the event that your BMI is 18.5 or less, we don't suggest that you leave on Stage 1 of the diet. In the event that your BMI is somewhere in the range of 18.5 and 20, we would at present urge alert, since following the diet may imply that your BMI falls underneath 18.5.

I'm corpulent—Is the Sirtfood Diet directly for me?

Indeed! Try not to be put off by the way that lone a little minority of the members who set out on our pilot study were corpulent. This is on the grounds that the pilot study was done in a wellbeing and wellness club where individuals are commonly fitter and more wellbeing cognizant. Rather, be prodded on by the way that the rare sorts of people who were corpulent had stunningly better outcomes than our healthy-weight members. These outcomes have been reproduced by a great many individuals who have attempted the diet in reality. In view of the investigation into sirtuin actuation, you ought to likewise remain to harvest the best changes in your prosperity. Being corpulent builds the danger of various incessant medical issues, yet these are the very sicknesses that Sirtfoods help to insure against.

I've Arrived at my objective Weight and Would Prefer not to Lose any More— Do I Quit Eating Sirtfoods?

In the first place, congrats on your weight-loss accomplishment! You've had incredible accomplishment with Sirtfoods, however, it doesn't end now. While we don't suggest further calorie limitation, your diet should in any case give sufficient Sirtfoods. A significant number of our customers are currently at their optimal body structure however keeping on eating Sirtfood-rich diets. The incredible thing about Sirtfoods is that they are a lifestyle. The most ideal approach to consider them with respect to weight the board is that they help carry the body to the weight and synthesis it was intended to be. From here, they work to keep up and keep you looking and feeling incredible.

I've Completed Stage 2—Do I Quit Drinking the Morning Sirtfood Green Squeeze Now?

The green juice is our preferred method to get an awesome hit of Sirtfoods to begin the day, so we embrace its drawn-out utilization. Our Sirtfood green juice was deliberately intended to incorporate fixings that give a full range of sirtuin-actuating supplements in powerful fat-consuming and prosperity boosting dosages. In any case, we are totally supportive of assortment, and keeping in mind that we do suggest you proceed with a morning juice, we completely bolster anybody hoping to try different things with various Sirtfood juice creations.

I Take Drug—Is it alright to Follow the Diet?

The Sirtfood Diet is appropriate for a great many people, but since of its ground-breaking consequences for fat consumption and wellbeing, it can change certain malady forms and the activities of prescription recommended by your primary care physician. In like manner, certain drugs are not reasonable in a fasting state. During the preliminary of the Sirtfood Diet, we surveyed the appropriateness of every individual before the person in question left on the diet, particularly the individuals who were taking prescription.

Would I Be Able to Follow the Diet in Case I'm pregnant?

We don't suggest leaving on the Sirtfood Diet on the off chance that you are attempting to consider or in the event that you are pregnant or breastfeeding. It is an incredible weight-loss diet, which makes it unacceptable. In any case, don't be put off eating a lot of Sirtfoods, since these are particularly healthy nourishments to incorporate as a component of a decent and differed diet for pregnancy. You will need to stay away from red wine, because of its liquor substance, and cutoff stimulated things, for example, espresso, green tea, and cocoa so as not to surpass 200 milligrams for each day of caffeine during pregnancy (one cup of moment espresso ordinarily contains around 100 milligrams of caffeine).

Is Sirtfoods appropriate for Youngsters?

The Sirtfood Diet is an amazing weight-loss diet and not intended for youngsters. In any case, that doesn't imply that youngsters should pass up the phenomenal medical advantages offered by incorporating more Sirtfoods in their general diet. A greater part of Sirtfoods speak to incredibly healthy nourishments for youngsters and assist them with accomplishing adjusted and nutritious diets. A large number of the plans intended for Stage 2 of the diet were made in light of families, including youngsters' taste buds. Any semblance of the Sirtfood pizza, the bean stew with meat, and the Sirtfood nibbles are flawless kid agreeable nourishments with a nutritional worth better than common food contributions for kids.

Will I Get a Migraine or Feel tired during Stage 1?

Stage 1 of the Sirtfood Diet gives incredible normally happening food mixes in sums that the vast majority would not get in their ordinary diet, and certain individuals can respond as they adjust to this sensational nutritional change. This can incorporate manifestations, for example, a gentle migraine or tiredness, despite the fact that we would say these impacts are minor and brief.

Obviously, if side effects are serious or give you purpose behind concern, we suggest you look for brief clinical counsel.

Would it Be a good Idea for me to Take Enhancements?

Except if explicitly endorsed for you by your primary care physician or other social insurance proficient, we don't suggest aimless utilization of nutritional enhancements. You will ingest a huge and synergistic cluster of characteristic plant mixes from Sirtfoods, and it is these that will benefit you. You can't repeat these advantages with nutritional enhancements and, truth be told, some nutritional enhancements, for example, cell reinforcements, particularly whenever taken at high portions, may really meddle with the helpful impacts of Sirtfoods, which is the exact opposite thing you need.

How regularly Would I Be Able to Rehash Stages 1 and 2?

Stage 1 can be rehashed on the off chance that you sense that you need a weight-loss or wellbeing help. To guarantee that there are no drawn-out negative impacts to your digestion from calorie limitation, you should hold up, in any event, a month prior to rehashing. Be that as it may, we really locate that the vast majority need to rehash it no more regularly than once like clockwork probably and keep on getting astounding outcomes. Rather, in the event that you find you've gone off course, need some new-tuning, or need more Sirtfood force, we suggest rehashing a few or the entire days of the Stage 2 area as regularly as you like. All things considered, Stage 2 is tied in with setting up a lifelong method of eating.

Does the Sirtfood Diet Give enough Fiber?

Numerous Sirtfoods are normally rich in fiber. Onions, endive, and pecans are striking sources, with buckwheat and Medjool dates truly sticking out, implying that a Sirtfood-rich diet doesn't miss the mark in the fiber office. In any event, during Stage 1, when food utilization is diminished, the greater part of us will at present be devouring a fiber amount we are utilized to, particularly on the off chance that we pick the plans that contain buckwheat, beans, and lentils from the menu choices.

I've Found out about Super Nourishments—Would it Be advisable for me to Incorporate these in my Diet as Well?

The main thing you have to think about the term superfood is that it's anything but a logical term at everything except a showcasing motto. You don't have to worry about supposed super nourishments on the grounds that the Sirtfood Diet unites the most advantageous food sources on earth into a progressive better approach for eating. Similarly, as it is a slip-up to depend on taking a straightforward nutrient pill to make us healthy, so too it is a mix-up to depend on a solitary superfood to do likewise. It is the entire diet, comprised of a wide range of Sirtfoods and their huge range of normal mixes, acting in cooperative energy that is the genuine mystery to accomplishing weight loss and lifelong wellbeing.

Do I Need to Do Stage 1 for Seven Days—Would I Be Able to Do less?

There's nothing otherworldly about Stage 1 being seven days. It is basically what we chose for our preliminary. We picked that since it was long enough to get amazing outcomes, however, not all that long that it got difficult. It likewise fits perfectly into individuals' lives. Seven days is what was tried and what is demonstrated to be compelling. In any case, if for reasons unknown, you find that you have to stop it by a day or two, do as such by finishing up to the finish of Day 5 or Day 6. Try not to stress; you will at present harvest a lot of the advantages.

Would I Be Able to Eat anything I Desire Once I Eat a Lot of Sirtfoods and still Get Results?

One of the key reasons the Sirtfood Diet works so well long haul is that it advances great food as opposed to deriding awful food. Diets of rejection basically don't work long haul. The facts confirm that handled nourishments that are high in sugars and fats lessen the sirtuin movement in the body, and in this manner, a high utilization will diminish the advantages of Sirtfoods. In any case, on the off chance that you maintain your emphasis on expending a diet rich in Sirtfoods, in our experience you will find that you are charmingly fulfilled and will have less want for those prepared nourishments and wind up devouring far less garbage than the normal individual accordingly.

Would I Be Able to Eat the same Number of Sirtfoods, even the unhealthy ones, as I Like and still Get Thinner?

Truly! Keep in mind, calories and the drive to tally them is present-day "headway." Over the way of life and incalculable ages that have profited by Sirtfoods, such an idea didn't exist, and they're basically was no need. Individuals ate as they felt like it, and remained thin and liberated from infection. Given Sirtfoods' consequences for managing digestion and hunger, you just don't have to stress over eating an excessive number of them.

While this isn't a solicitation to everything you-can-eat challenge, don't hesitate to eat as much Sirtfood as you like to fulfill your regular hunger. Our one special case is Medjool dates.

Chapter 7- Breakfast

1. Creamy Strawberry & Cherry Smoothie

Preparation Time: 10 minutes

Cooking Time: 15 minutes

Servings: 1

Ingredients:

- 3½ ounces strawberries

- 3 ounces frozen pitted cherries

- 1 tablespoon plain full-fat yogurt

- 6 ounces unsweetened soya milk

Directions:

Place the ingredients into a blender then process until smooth. Serve and enjoy.

Nutrition: Calories: 132, Carbs: 46 grams, Fat: 3 grams, Protein: 24 grams

2. Strawberry & Citrus Blend

Preparation Time: 10 minutes

Cooking Time: 15 minutes

Servings: 1

Ingredients:

- 3 ounces strawberries

- 1 apple, cored

- 1 orange, peeled

- ½ avocado, peeled and de-stoned

- ½ teaspoon matcha powder

- 1 lime juice

Directions:

Place ingredients into a blender with enough water to cover them and process until smooth.

Nutrition: Calories: 272, Carbs: 3 grams, Fat: 2 grams, Protein: 25 grams

3. Grapefruit & Celery Blast

Preparation Time: 10 minutes

Cooking Time: 15 minutes

Servings: 1

Ingredients:

- 1 grapefruit, peeled

- 2 stalks of celery

- 2 ounces kale

- ½ teaspoon matcha powder

Directions:

Place ingredients into a blender with water to cover them and blitz until smooth.

Nutrition: Calories: 71, Carbs: 16 grams, Fat: 0 gram, Protein: 2 grams

4. Orange & Celery Crush

Preparation Time: 10 minutes

Cooking Time: 15 minutes

Servings: 1

Ingredients:

- 1 carrot, peeled

- 3 stalks of celery

- 1 orange, peeled

- ½ teaspoon matcha powder

- Juice of 1 lime

Directions:

Place ingredients into a blender with enough water to cover them and blitz until smooth.

Nutrition: Calories: 95, Carbs: 70 grams, Fat: 0 gram, Protein: 0 gram

5. Tropical Chocolate Delight

Preparation Time: 10 minutes

Cooking Time: 15 minutes

Servings: 1

Ingredients:

- 1 mango, peeled & de-stoned

- 3 ounces fresh pineapple, chopped

- 2 ounces kale

- 1 ounce rocket

- 1 tablespoon 100% cocoa powder or cacao nibs

- 5 ounces of coconut milk

Directions:

Place ingredients into a blender and blitz until smooth. You can add a little water if it seems too thick.

Nutrition: Calories: 427, Carbs: 56 grams, Fat: 0 gram, Protein: 0 gram

6. Walnut & Spiced Apple Tonic

Preparation Time: 10 minutes

Cooking Time: 15 minutes

Servings: 1

Ingredients:

- 6 walnuts halves

- 1 apple, cored

- 1 banana

- ½ teaspoon matcha powder

- ½ teaspoon cinnamon

- Pinch of ground nutmeg

Directions:

Place ingredients into a blender and add sufficient water to cover them. Blitz until smooth and creamy.

Nutrition: Calories: 95, Carbs: 12 grams, Fat: 0 gram, Protein: 0 gram

7. Mushroom Scramble Eggs

Preparation Time: 10 minutes

Cooking Time: 15 minutes

Servings: 1

Ingredients:

- 2 Eggs

- 1 teaspoon curry powder

- 1teaspoon ground turmeric

- 1teaspoon olive oil, extra virgin

- 4 teaspoons chopped kale

- Handful mushroom sliced

- 1 teaspoon chopped parsley

- Seeds mixture or rooster sauce as a topper (optional)

Directions:

Start with making the paste of curry powder, water and turmeric.

After that start steaming kale for 2-3 minutes only.

Then heat the olive oil in a pan and start frying the mushrooms with chilies until they become brown.

Now, whisk the eggs and mix them in curry, turmeric paste and cook with kale by using medium heat.

Now, garnish with parsley and enjoy it.

Nutrition: Calories: 347, Carbs: 4 grams, Fat: 21 grams, Protein: 33 grams

8. Sirt Green Diet Juice

Preparation Time: 10 minutes

Cooking Time: 0 minute

Servings: 1

Ingredients:

- 1 teaspoon Parsley

- Handful or 6 teaspoons arugula

- 2 handful or 5 tablespoons kale

- 2-3 stalks or 10 tablespoons green celery

- Half green apple

- Half lemon juiced form

- ½ teaspoon matcha powder

Directions:

Gather the entire ingredients and put them in a blender, blend it well until it becomes juice now garnish it and enjoy

Nutrition: Calories: 37, Carbs: 11 grams, Fat: 1 gram, Protein: 5 grams

9. Chia Breakfast Bowl

Preparation Time: 10 minutes

Cooking Time: 0 minute

Servings:

Ingredients:

- 1-3 teaspoon chia seeds

- 2/3 cup nut milk (almond or coconut)

- A pinch of salt

- Maple syrup, honey or nectar to taste

- Coconut flakes or seasonal fruit like blueberries as a topper

Directions:

Start with mixing the chia seeds in almond milk and continue to stir them efficiently,

After let the seeds sit for approximately 12 minutes until they become completely swollen.

In the end, put the honey, fruit you want and very little salt. Now enjoy and serve.

Nutrition: Calories: 220, Carbs: 25 grams, Fat: 11 grams, Protein: 8 grams

10.   Tofu Berry Smoothie

Preparation Time: 5 minutes

Cooking Time:

Servings: 1

Ingredients:

- 6 ounces silken tofu

- 2/3 cup soy milk

- 1 tablespoon honey

- 1 medium-sized banana

- 1 cup fresh blueberries

- Ice cubes optional

Directions:

Start with removing water from tofu, now gather the ingredients.

In a blender, put banana, tofu and soy milk to blend for 40 sec.

Now, put blueberries and start blending again until turns smooth.

In the end, put the ice cubes, rest of berries and honey and blend a little again

Now, serve and enjoy.

Nutrition: Calories: 157, Carbs: 33 grams, Fat: 2 grams, Protein: 4 grams

11.   Sirt Food Cocktail

Preparation Time: 5 minutes

Cooking Time: 0 minute

Servings: 1

Ingredients:

- 3 ounces kale

- 2 ounces strawberries

- 1 apple, cored

- 2 sticks of celery

- 1 tablespoon parsley

- 1 teaspoon of matcha powder

- Squeeze lemon juice (optional) to taste

Directions:

Place the ingredients into a blender and add enough water to cover the ingredients and blitz to a smooth consistency.

Nutrition: Calories: 101, Carbs: 12 grams, Fat: 1 gram, Protein: 10 grams

12.   Summer Berry Smoothie

Preparation Time: 10 minutes

Cooking Time: 0 minute

Servings: 1

Ingredients:

- 2 ounces blueberries

- 2 ounces strawberries

- 1 ounce blackcurrants

- 1 ounce red grapes

- 1 carrot, peeled

- 1 orange, peeled

- Juice of 1 lime

Directions:

Place all of the ingredients into a blender and cover them with water. Blitz until smooth. You can also add some crushed ice and a mint leaf to garnish.

Nutrition: Calories: 146, Carbs: 0 gram, Fat: 7 grams, Protein: 19 grams

13.   Mango, Celery & Ginger Smoothie

Preparation Time: 5 minutes

Cooking Time: 0 minute

Servings: 1

Ingredients:

- 1 stalk of celery

- 2 ounces kale

- 1 apple, cored

- 2 ounces mango, peeled, de-stoned and chopped

- 1 inch chunk of fresh ginger root, peeled and chopped

Directions:

Put all the ingredients into a blender with some water and blitz until smooth. Add ice to make your smoothie really refreshing.

Nutrition: Calories: 105, Carbs: 35 grams, Fat: 1 gram, Protein: 13 grams

Chapter 8 - Main Meals

1. Coq Au Vin

Preparation Time: 10 minutes

Cooking Time: 15 minutes

Servings: 8

Ingredients:

- 16 ounces button mushrooms

- 3½ ounces streaky bacon, chopped

- 16 chicken thighs, skin removed

- 3 cloves of garlic, crushed

- 3 tablespoons fresh parsley, chopped

- 3 carrots, chopped

- 2 red onions, chopped

- 2 tablespoons plain flour

- 2 tablespoons olive oil

- 750mls 1¼ pints red wine

- 1 bouquet grain

Directions:

On a large plate, put the flour and coat the chicken in it. Heat the olive oil then add the chicken and brown it, before setting aside. Fry the bacon in the pan then add the onion and cook for 5 minutes. Pour in the red wine and add the chicken, carrots, bouquet grain and garlic. Transfer it to a large ovenproof dish. Cook at 180C/360F for an hour. Remove the bouquet grain and skim off any excess fat, if necessary. Add in the mushrooms and cook for 15 minutes. Stir in the parsley just before serving.

Nutrition: Calories: 459, Carbs: 9 grams, Fat: 21 grams, Protein: 46 grams

2. Turkey Satay Skewers

Preparation Time: 10 minutes

Cooking Time: 15 minutes

Servings: 2

Ingredients:

- 9 ounces turkey breast, cubed

- 1 ounce smooth peanut butter

- 1 clove of garlic, crushed

- ½ small bird's eye chili or more if you like it hotter, finely chopped

- ½ teaspoon ground turmeric

- 7 ounces of coconut milk

- 2 teaspoons soy sauce

Directions:

Combine the coconut milk, peanut butter, turmeric, soy sauce, garlic and chili. Add the turkey pieces to the bowl and stir them until they are completely coated. Push the turkey onto metal skewers. Place the satay skewers on a barbeque or under a hot grill broiler and cook for 4-5 minutes on each side, until they are completely cooked.

Nutrition: Calories: 431,Carbs: 17 grams, Fat: 2 grams, Protein: 30 grams

3. Salmon & Capers

Preparation Time: 10 minutes

Cooking Time: 15 minutes

Servings: 4

Ingredients:

- 3 ounces Greek yogurt

- 4 salmon fillets, skin removed

- 4 teaspoons Dijon Mustard

- 1 tablespoon capers, chopped

- 2 teaspoons fresh parsley

- Zest of 1 lemon

Directions:

Put the yogurt, mustard, lemon zest, parsley and capers in a mixing bowl. Thoroughly coat the salmon in the mixture. Place the salmon under a hot grill broiler and cook for 3-4 minutes on each side, or until the fish is cooked. Serve with mashed potatoes and vegetables or a large green leafy salad.

Nutrition: Calories: 321, Carbs: 12 grams, Fat: 26 grams, Protein: 32 grams

4. Moroccan Chicken Casserole

Preparation Time: 10 minutes

Cooking Time: 15 minutes

Servings: 4

Ingredients:

- 9 ounces tinned chickpeas garbanzo beans drained

- 4 chicken breasts, cubed

- 4 Medrol dates, halved

- 6 dried apricots, halved

- 1 red onion, sliced

- 1 carrot, chopped

- 1 teaspoon ground cumin

- 1 teaspoon ground cinnamon

- 1 teaspoon ground turmeric

- 1 bird's-eye chili, chopped

- 1 pint chicken stock broth

- 1 ounce cornflour

- 2 ounces of water

- 2 tablespoons fresh coriander

Directions:

Place the chicken, chickpeas garbanzo beans, onion, carrot, chili, cumin, turmeric, cinnamon and stock broth into a large saucepan. Put it to the boil, and reduce heat after that simmer for 25 minutes. Add in the dates and apricots and simmer for 10 minutes. In a cup, mix the cornflour together with the water until it becomes a smooth paste. Pour the mixture into the saucepan and stir until it thickens. Add in the coriander cilantro and mix well. Serve with buckwheat or couscous.

Nutrition: Calories: 401, Carbs: 0 gram, Fat: 13 grams, Protein: 39 grams

5. Chili Con Carne

Preparation Time: 10 minutes

Cooking Time: 15 minutes

Servings: 4

Ingredients:

- 16 ounces lean minced beef

- 14 ounces chopped tomatoes

- 7 ounces red kidney beans

- 2 tablespoons tomato purée

- 2 cloves of garlic, crushed

- 2 red onions, chopped

- 2 bird's-eye chilies, finely chopped

- 1 red pepper bell pepper, chopped

- 1 stick of celery, finely chopped

- 1 tablespoon cumin

- 1 tablespoon turmeric

- 1 tablespoon cocoa powder

- 14 ounces beef stock broth

- 6 ounces red wine

- 1 tablespoon olive oil

Directions:

Put the oil in a saucepan then add the onion and cook for 5 minutes. Add in the garlic, celery, chili, turmeric, and cumin and cook for 2 minutes before adding then meat then cook for another 5 minutes. Pour in the stock broth, red wine, tomatoes, tomato purée, red pepper bell pepper, kidney beans and cocoa powder. Let it simmer for 45 minutes, keep it covered and stirring occasionally. Serve with brown rice or buckwheat.

Nutrition: Calories: 390, Carbs: 18 grams, Fat: 22 grams, Protein: 25 grams

6. Prawn & Coconut Curry

Preparation Time: 10 minutes

Cooking Time: 15 minutes

Servings: 4

Ingredients:

- 14 ounces tinned chopped tomatoes

- 14 ounces large prawns shrimps, shelled and raw

- 1 ounce fresh coriander cilantro chopped

- 3 red onions, finely chopped

- 3 cloves of garlic, crushed

- 2 bird's eye chilies

- ½ teaspoon ground coriander cilantro

- ½ teaspoon turmeric

- 14 ounces of coconut milk

- 1 tablespoon olive oil

- Juice of 1 lime

Directions:

Place the onions, garlic, tomatoes, chilies, lime juice, turmeric, ground coriander, chilies and half of the fresh coriander cilantro into a blender and blitz until you have a smooth curry paste. In a frying pan, put the oil, add the pasta and cook for 2 minutes. Stir in the coconut milk and warm it thoroughly. Add the prawn's shrimps to the paste and cook them until they have turned pink and are completely cooked. Stir in the fresh coriander cilantro. Serve with rice.

Nutrition: Calories:322,Carbs: 7 grams, Fat: 27 grams, Protein: 15 grams

7. Turmeric Sautéed Greens

Preparation Time: 3 minutes

Cooking Time: 5 minutes

Servings: 3-4

Ingredients:

- 1 tablespoon olive oil

- 1 2-inch piece fresh turmeric

- ¼ teaspoon kosher salt

- 3 garlic cloves, minced

- 2 tablespoons water

- 2 bunches kale, spinach, or Swiss chard, thinly sliced

Directions:

Firstly, heat oil in a large saucepan by using medium heat.

Now, add garlic and turmeric and sauté for 30 seconds.

Further, add kale and salt and sauté for 1 minute.

At the last add water to the pan and cook stirring until the greens are just wilted and serve.

Nutrition: Calories: 60, Carbs: 9 grams, Fat: 3 grams, Protein: 3 grams

8. Cauliflower rice

Preparation Time: 10 minutes

Cooking Time: 15 minutes

Servings: 2

Ingredients:

- 2 tablespoons olive oil

- 1 yellow or orange bell pepper, seeded and diced

- 1 head cauliflower, chopped in the food processor until it resembles rice

- 1 onion, finely diced

- 3 cups fresh spinach, roughly chopped

- 1 cup shelled edamame

- ½ teaspoon kosher salt

- 2 teaspoons fresh ginger, minced

- 3 tablespoons low sodium soy sauce

- 2 scallions, chopped

Directions:

Firstly, heat a large wok or sauté pan over medium heat, add oil and sauté onion and ginger for 1 minute. Put bell pepper and cook for 1 minute.

Now, add the cauliflower and cook for an additional 2-3 minutes. Add spinach, edamame, soy sauce and salt. Cook for 3-4 minutes or until cauliflower is tender.

Finely, top with chopped scallions and serve.

Nutrition: Calories: 62, Carbs: 5 grams, Fat: 4 grams, Protein: 2 grams

9. Seafood Stew

Preparation time: 15 minutes

Cooking Time: 40 minutes

Servings: 4-6

Ingredients:

- 1 tablespoon oil
- 6 garlic cloves, minced
- 1 teaspoon kosher salt
- 1 cup dry white wine
- 1 large onion, diced
- 1 bay leaf
- 28ounces can diced tomatoes
- ½ pound clams
- ½ pound shrimp, peeled and deveined
- ½ pound shrimp, peeled and deveined
- 1 cup clam juice
- ½ pound mussels
- ¼ cup minced parsley, for garnish, optional

Directions:

Take a large pot, heat oil by using medium heat.

Put the onions and cook for 3-4 minutes, until tender. Add garlic and sauté for another minute.

Now, add the wine, tomatoes, clam juice, bay leaf and salt. Bring to a boil, then reduce heat to medium and simmer for 20 minutes.

Further, put in all the seafood at once and stir to combine. Cook until shrimp is pink and cooked through and mussels and clams have opened about 5-7 minutes.

Finely, Garnish with parsley if desired and serve immediately

Nutrition: Calories: 177, Carbs: 15 grams, Fat: 4 grams, Protein: 21 grams

10.   Sautéed Collard Greens

Preparation time: 5 minutes

Cooking Time: 25 minutes

Servings: 4

Ingredients:

- 1 slice thick-cut bacon, diced

- 1 bunch collard greens

- 2 garlic cloves, minced

- ½ teaspoon kosher salt

Directions:

Firstly, Put the bacon in a sauté pan over medium-low heat and cook for 5 minutes to render as fatter as possible.

While the bacon is cooking, remove the stems from the collard greens, and thinly slice the leaves across.

Now, add the garlic to the pan and cook for 1 minute. Add the greens and salt, stir well to coat the greens with the bacon fat, reduce heat to low, and cook for 5 minutes, until wilted, stirring occasionally. If you like them softer, cook for 10 minutes.

Nutrition: Calories: 39, Carbs: 7 grams, Fat: 1 gram, Protein: 3 grams

11.   Mussels in Red Wine Sauce

Preparation Time: 10 minutes

Cooking Time: 10 minutes

Servings: 2

Ingredients:

- 32 ounces mussels

- 14 ounces tins of chopped tomatoes

- 1 ounces butter

- 1 tablespoon fresh chives, chopped

- 1 tablespoon fresh parsley, chopped

- 1 bird's-eye chili, finely chopped

- 4 cloves of garlic, crushed

- 14 ounces red wine

- Juice of 1 lemon

Directions:

Wash the mussels, remove their beards and set them aside. Heat the butter in a large saucepan and add in the red wine. Reduce the heat and add the parsley, chives, chilli and garlic whilst stirring. Add in the tomatoes, lemon juice and mussels. Cover the saucepan and cook for 2-3.Remove the saucepan from the heat and take out any mussels which haven't opened and discard them. Serve and eat immediately.

Nutrition: Calories: 364, Carbs: 26 grams, Fat: 12 grams, Protein: 32 grams

12. Tomato & Goat's Cheese Pizza

Preparation Time: 10 minutes

Cooking Time: 25 minutes

Servings: 2

Ingredients:

- 8 ounces buckwheat flour

- 2 teaspoons dried yeast

- Pinch of salt

- 15 ounces slightly water

- 1 teaspoon olive oil

For the Topping:

- 3 ounces feta cheese, crumbled

- 3 ounces passata (or tomato paste)

- 1 tomato, sliced

- 1 red onion, finely chopped

- 1 ounce rocket (arugula) leaves, chopped

Directions:

In a bowl, combine all the ingredients for the pizza dough then allow it to stand for at least an hour until it has doubled in size. Roll the dough out to a size to suit you. Spoon the passata onto the base and add the rest of the toppings.

Bake in the oven at 200C/400F for 15-20 minutes or until browned at the edges and crispy and serve.

Nutrition: Calories: 562, Carbs: 50 grams, Fat: 16 grams, Protein: 16 grams

13.   Tofu Thai Curry

Preparation Time: 10 minutes

Cooking Time: 20 minutes

Servings: 4

Ingredients:

- 14 ounces tofu, diced

- 7 ounces sugar snap peas

- 2 inches chunk fresh ginger root, peeled and finely chopped

- 2 red onions, chopped

- 2 cloves of garlic, crushed

- 2 bird's eye chilies

- 2 tablespoons tomato puree

- 1 stalk of lemongrass, inner stalks only

- 1 tablespoon fresh coriander (cilantro), chopped

- 1 teaspoon cumin

- ½ pint coconut milk

- 7 ounces vegetable stock (broth)

- 1 tablespoon virgin olive oil

- Juice of 1 lime

Directions:

Heat the oil in a frying pan, add the onion and cook for 4 minutes. Add in the chillies, cumin, ginger, and garlic and cook for 2 minutes. Add the tomato puree, lemongrass, sugar snap peas, lime juice and tofu and cook for 2 minutes. Pour in the stock (broth), coconut milk and coriander (cilantro) and simmer for 5 minutes. Serve with brown rice or buckwheat and a handful of rocket (arugula) leaves on the side.

Nutrition: Calories: 270, Carbs: 26 grams, Fat: 11 grams, Protein: 22 grams

Chapter 9 - Snacks Recipe

1. Lemon Ricotta Cookies with Lemon Glaze

Preparation Time: 10 minutes

Cooking Time: 1 hour

Servings: 8

- 2 ½ cups all-purpose flour

- 1 teaspoon baking powder

- 1 teaspoon salt

- 1 tablespoon unsalted butter softened

- 2 cups of sugar

- 2 capsules

- 1 teaspoon (15-ounce) container whole-milk ricotta cheese

- 3 tablespoons lemon juice

- 1 lemon, zested

Glaze:

- 1 ½ cups powdered sugar

- 3tablespoons lemon juice

- 1 lemon, zested

Directions:

- Preheat the oven to 375 degrees F.

- At a medium bowl, combine the flour, baking powder, and salt. set aside.

- From the big bowl, blend the butter and the sugar levels. With an electric mixer, beat the sugar and butter until light and fluffy, about three minutes. Add the eggs1 at a time, beating until incorporated.

- Insert the ricotta cheese, lemon juice, and lemon zest. Beat to blend. Stir in the dry skin.

- Line two baking sheets with parchment paper. Spoon the dough (approximately 2 tablespoons of each cookie) on the baking sheets. Bake for fifteen minutes, until slightly golden at the borders. Remove from the oven and allow the biscuits remaining baking sheet for about 20 minutes.

Glaze:

Combine the powdered sugar lemon juice and lemon peel in a small bowl and then stir until smooth. Spoon approximately 1/2-tsp on each cookie and make use of the back of the spoon to lightly disperse. Allow glaze harden for approximately two hours. Pack the biscuits to a decorative jar.

Nutrition: Calories 113, Fat 3.5 grams, Carbs 19 grams, Protein 2 grams

2. Home-Made Marshmallow Fluff

Preparation Time: 5 minutes

Cooking Time: 1 hour 30 minutes

Servings: 3

Ingredients:

- ¾ cup of sugar

- ½ cup light corn syrup

- ¼ cup of water

- ⅛ Teaspoon salt

- 3 little egg whites

- ¼ teaspoon cream of tartar

- 1 ½ teaspoon vanilla infusion

Directions:

In a little pan, mix together sugar, corn syrup, salt, and water. Attach a candy thermometer into the side of this pan, which makes sure it will not touch the underside of the pan. Set aside.

From the bowl of a stand mixer, combine egg whites and cream of tartar. Begin to whip on medium speed with the whisk attachment.

Meanwhile, turn the burner on top and place the pan with the sugar mix onto heat. Allow mix into a boil and heat to 240 degrees, stirring periodically.

The aim is to find the egg whites whipped to soft peaks and also the sugar heated to 240 degrees at near the same moment. Simply stop stirring the egg whites once they hit soft peaks.

Once the sugar has already reached 240 amounts, turn noodle onto reducing. Insert a little quantity of the popular sugar mix and let it mix. Insert still another little sum of the sugar mix. Carry on to add mix slowly, and that means you never scramble the egg whites.

After all of the sugar was added into the egg whites, then turn the rate of this mixer and also keep to overcome concoction for around 79 minutes until the fluff remains glossy and stiff. In roughly the 5 minute mark, then add vanilla extract.

Use fluff immediately or store in an airtight container in the fridge for around two weeks.

Nutrition: Calories 322, Fat 0.3 grams, Carbs, 79 grams, Protein 0.8 grams

3. Guilt totally free Banana Icecream

Preparation Time: 5 minutes

Cooking Time: 0 minute

Servings: 2

Ingredients:

- 3 quite ripe banana - peeled and rooted

- A couple of chocolate chips

- 2 tablespoons skim milk

Directions:

- Throw all ingredients into a food processor and blend until creamy.

- Eat freeze and appreciate afterward.

Nutrition: Calories: 210, Protein: 3 grams, Carbs: 54 grams, Fat: 0.8 grams

4. Perfect little PB Snack Balls

Preparation Time: 5 minutes

Cooking Time: 0 minute

Servings: 2

Ingredients:

- ½ cup chunky peanut butter

- 3 tablespoons flax seeds

- 3 tablespoons wheat germ

- 1 tablespoon honey or agave

- ¼ cup powder

Directions:

Blend dry ingredients and adding from the honey and peanut butter.

Mix well and roll into chunks and then conclude by rolling into wheat germ.

Nutrition: Calories 103.1, Fat 4.3 grams, Carbs 15.4 grams, Protein 2.3 grams

5. Dark Chocolate Pretzel Cookies

Preparation Time: 10 minutes

Cooking Time: 20 minutes

Servings: 6

Ingredients:

- 1 cup yogurt

- ½ teaspoon baking soda

- ¼ teaspoon salt

- ¼ teaspoon cinnamon

- 4 tablespoons butter softened

- 1/3 cup brown sugar

- 1 egg

- 2 teaspoons vanilla

- ½ cup dark chocolate chips

- ½ cup pretzels chopped

Directions:

- Pre Heat oven to 350 degrees.

- At a medium bowl, whisk together the sugar, butter, vanilla, and egg.

- In another bowl, stir together the flour, baking soda, and salt.

- Stir the bread mixture in using all the moist components, along with the chocolate chips and pretzels until just blended.

- Drop a large spoonful of dough on an unlined baking sheet.

- Bake for 15-17 minutes, or until the bottoms are somewhat all crispy.

- Allow cooling on a wire rack.

Nutrition: Calories: 190, Fat: 8 grams, Carbs: 28 grams, Protein: 2 grams

6. Mascarpone Cheesecake with Almond Crust

Preparation Time: 15 minutes

Cooking Time: 1 hour 30 minutes

Servings: 8

Ingredients:

Crust

- ½ cup slivered almonds

- 8 teaspoons or 2/3 cup graham cracker crumbs

- 2 tablespoons sugar

- 1tablespoon salted butter melted

Filling

- 1 (8-ounce) packages cream cheese, room temperature

- 1 (8-ounce) container mascarpone cheese, room temperature

- ¾ cup of sugar

- 1 teaspoon fresh lemon juice (I needed to use imitation Lemon-juice)

- 1 teaspoon

- 2 large eggs, room temperature

Directions:

- **For the crust:** Preheat oven to 350 degrees F. Take per 9-inch diameter around the pan (I had a throw off). Finely grind the almonds, cracker crumbs sugar in a food processor or (I used my magic bullet). Bring the butter and process until moist crumbs form.

Press the almond mixture on the base of the prepared pan (maybe not on the surfaces of the pan). Bake the crust until its put and start to brown, about 1-2 minutes. Cool. Decrease the oven temperature to 325 degrees F.

- **For your filling:** With an electric mixer, beat the cream cheese, mascarpone cheese, and sugar in a large bowl until smooth, occasionally scraping down the sides of the jar using a rubber spatula. Beat in the lemon juice and vanilla. Add the eggs1 at a time, beating until combined after each addition.

Pour the cheese mixture on the crust from the pan. Put the pan into a big skillet or Pyrex dish Pour enough hot water to the roasting pan to come halfway up, the sides of one's skillet. Bake until the middle of this racket goes slightly when the pan is gently shaken, about 1 hour (the dessert will get business if it's cold). Transfer the cake to a stand; trendy for 1 hour. Refrigerate before the cheesecake is cold, at least eight hours.

- **Topping**: Squeezed just a small thick cream at the microwave using a busted up Lindt chocolate brown -- afterward, the got a Ziploc baggie and cut out a hole at the corner then poured the melted chocolate to the baggie and used this to decorate the cake.

Nutrition: Calories: 410, Fat: 26 grams, Carbs: 39 grams, Protein: 7 grams

7. Marshmallow Pop Corn Balls

Preparation Time: 5 minutes

Cooking Time: 10 minutes

Servings: 4

Ingredients:

- 2 bag of microwave popcorn

- 1 12.6 ounces. Tote M&M's

- 3 cups honey roasted peanuts

- 1 pkg. 16 ounce. Massive marshmallows

- 1 cup butter, cubed

Directions:

- In a bowl, blend the popcorn, peanuts and M&M's.

- In a big pot, combine marshmallows and butter.

- Cook medium-low warmth.

- Insert popcorn mix, blend nicely

- Spray muffin tins with nonstop cooking spray.

- When cool enough to handle, spray hands together with nonstick cooking spray and then shape into chunks and put into a muffin tin to carry contour.

- Add Popsicle stick into each chunk and then let cool.

- Wrap each person in vinyl when chilled.

Nutrition: Calories: 150, Fat: 0 gram, Carbs: 35 grams, Protein: 2 grams

8. Home-made Ice-cream Drumsticks

Preparation Time: 10 minutes

Cooking Time: 0 minute

Servings: 8

Ingredients:

- Vanilla ice cream

- 2 Lindt Hazel Nut chunks

- Magical shell - out chocolate

- Sugar levels

- Nuts (I mixed crushed peppers and unsalted peanuts)

- Parchment newspaper

Directions:

- Soften ice cream and mixing topping - I had two sliced Lindt hazel nutballs.

- Fill underside of sugar with magic and nuts shell and top with ice cream.

- Wrap parchment paper round cone and then fill cone over about 1.5 inches across the cap of the cone (the newspaper can help to carry its shape).

- Shirt with magical nuts and shells.

- Freeze for about 20 minutes before the ice cream is business.

Nutrition: Calories: 299, Fat: 33 grams, Carbs: 16 grams, Protein: 7 grams

9. Ultimate Chocolate Chip Cookie n' Oreo Fudge Brownie Bar

Preparation Time: 15 minutes

Cooking Time: 1 hour

Servings: 8

Ingredients:

- 1 cup (2 sticks) butter, softened

- 1 cup granulated sugar

- ¾ cup light brown sugar

- 2 big egg

- 1 tablespoon pure vanilla extract

- 2 ½ cups all-purpose flour

- 1 teaspoon baking soda

- 1 teaspoon lemon

- 2 cups (12 ounces) milk chocolate chips

- 1 package Double Stuffed Oreos

- 1 Family-size (9×1 3) Brownie mixture

- ¼ cup hot fudge topping

Directions:

- Pre Heat oven to 350 degrees F.

- Cream the butter and sugars in a large bowl using an electric mixer at medium speed for 35 minutes.

- Add the vanilla and eggs and mix well to thoroughly combine. In another bowl, whisk together the flour, baking soda and salt, and slowly incorporate in the mixer till the bread is simply combined.

- Stir in chocolate chips.

- Spread the cookie dough at the bottom of a 9×1-3 baking dish that is wrapped with wax nonstick then coated with cooking spray.

- Cloth with a coating of Oreos. Mix together brownie mix, adding an optional 1/4 cup of hot fudge directly into the mixture.

- Twist the brownie batter within the Cookie-dough and Oreos.

- Cover with foil and bake at 350 degrees F for half an hour.

- Remove foil and continue baking for another 15 25 minutes.

- Let cool before cutting on brownies might nevertheless be gooey at the midst while warm, but will also, place up perfectly once chilled.

Nutrition: Calories: 483, Fat: 25 grams, Carbs: 64 grams, Protein: 5 grams

10.   Crunchy Chocolate Chip Coconut Macadamia Nut Cookies

Preparation Time: 10 minutes

Cooking Time: 10 minutes

Servings: 8

Ingredients:

* 1 cup yogurt

* ½ teaspoon baking soda

* ½ teaspoon salt

* 1 tablespoon of butter, softened

* 1 cup firmly packed brown sugar

* ½ cup of sugar

* 1 big egg

* ½ cup Semi-Sweet chocolate chips

* ½ cup sweetened flaked coconut

* ½ cup coarsely chopped dry-roasted the macadamia nuts

* ½ cup raisins

Directions:

* Preheat the oven to 325ºF.

- In a little bowl, whisk together the flour, oats and baking soda, and salt then places aside.

- On your mixer bowl, then mix together the butter/ sugar/egg mix.

- Mix from the flour/oats mix until just combined and stir into the chocolate chips, raisins, nuts, and coconut.

- Decked outsized bits on a parchment-lined cookie sheet.

- Bake for 1-3 minutes before biscuits are only barely golden brown.

- Remove from the oven and then leave the cookie sheets to cool at least 10 minutes.

Nutrition: Calories: 110, Fat: 6 grams, Carbs: 18 grams, Protein: 0 gram

11.   Pizza Kale Chips

Preparation Time: 10 minutes

Cooking Time: 20 minutes

Servings: 6

Ingredients:

- 9 ounces kale, chopped
- 2 ounces ground almonds
- 2 ounces Parmesan cheese
- 3 tablespoons tomato purée (tomato paste)
- ½ teaspoon mixed herbs
- ½ teaspoon oregano
- ½ teaspoon onion powder
- 2 tablespoons olive oil
- 3 ½ ounces water

Directions:

Place all of the ingredients, except the KALE, into the food processor and process until finely chopped into a smooth consistency. Toss the kale leaves in the Parmesan mixture, coating it really well. Spread the kale out onto 2 baking sheets. Bake in the oven at 170C/325F for 15 minutes, until crispy.

Nutrition: Calories: 149, Carbs: 18 grams, Fat: 10 grams, Protein: 11 grams,

12.   Rosemary & Garlic Kale Chips

Preparation Time: 10 minutes

Cooking Time: 40 minutes

Servings: 4

Ingredients:

- 9 ounces kale chips, chopped

- 2 sprigs of rosemary

- 2 clove of garlic

- 2 tablespoons olive oil

- Sea salt

- Freshly ground black pepper

Directions:

Gently warm the olive oil, rosemary and garlic over low heat for 10 minutes. Remove it from the heat and set aside to cool. Take the rosemary and garlic out of the oil and discard them. Toss the kale leaves in the oil making sure they are well coated. Season with salt and pepper. Spread the kale leaves onto 2 baking sheets and bake them in the oven at 170C/325F for 15 minutes, until crispy.

Nutrition: Calories: 55, Carbs: 8 grams, Fat: 9 grams, Protein: 5 grams

13.   Honey Chilli Nuts

Preparation Time: 5 minutes

Cooking Time: 15 minutes

Servings: 20

Ingredients:

- 5 ounces walnuts

- 5 ounces pecan nuts

- 2 ounces softened butter

- 1 tablespoon honey

- ½ bird's-eye chilli, very finely chopped and de-seeded

Directions:

Preheat the oven to 180C/360F. Combine the butter, honey and chilli in a bowl then add the nuts and stir them well. Spread the nuts onto a lined baking sheet and roast them in the oven for 10 minutes, stirring once halfway through. Remove from the oven and allow them to cool before eating.

Nutrition: Calories: 126, Carbs: 5 grams, Fat: 22 grams, Protein: 12 grams

Chapter 10 - Celebrities who Follow the Sirtfood Diet

Lorraine Pascale

Lorraine Pascale is probably the world's most well-known and well-praised chef and food enthusiast. She belongs to the United Kingdom, the same country in which the sirtfood diet was first introduced. She is known as a successful supermodel when Lorraine was sixteen years old. She took care of her chronically ill mother for many years, and it was the time when she found the importance of some particular foods in the nourishment of chronically ill patients. This turned her interests in entirely different directions. She started taking an interest in cooking, and in no time, she was recognized as the most well-known and widely praised chef of the world. She has written many books on diet and foods. Over one million copies of her books were sold solely in the UK, and this a huge success indeed. She is a TV host, and her shows are aired in more than 70 countries globally. The ratings of her shows are insane, and she is the most-watched chef globally.

The praise of the sirtfood diet from the guru herself was a significant breakthrough in the popularity of this dieting regime. She mentioned that the sirtfood diet is the best-known diet for her with thousands of benefits. She considers herself as the biggest fan of the sirtfood diet, which is enough with respect to the sirtfood diet. She mentioned that the sirtfood diet was a breakthrough in achieving the best shape of her life; even this person is a supermodel herself. So notably, these statements from the Lorraine Pascale are enough to establish the health benefits of the sirtfood diet.

David Haye

He is one of the most dynamic boxers in history. He belongs to the UK, and he has won many titles of boxing championships. He has fought for two different weight classes in the same year and won both titles as the world's champion, thanks to the sirtfood diet and his fantastic training. David Haye is a vegan who loves vegan foods. He also holds a company that makes vegan protein powders. The number one problem of different fat loss diets is the issue related to vegan followers. Most of the ordinary fat loss diets involve a high protein diet coming from the animal source, which is, of course, big trouble for vegan lovers. Some fat loss diets are also designed for vegans, and these diets don't have any space for the meat lovers. So this cross completion between vegan and non-vegan interest causes many issues for both categories. The sirtfood diet is unique in this regard. It contains a great variety of vegan foods as well as a perfect space for meat lovers. The diet can be modified according to personal interest, and it is a win-win situation for both. The consumer just has to stick with the basic principles of the sirtfood diet, which are very simple to follow.

This perfect diet for vegans provided significant benefits to vegan boxer David Haye during his competitions. He mentioned that the sirtfood diet provided him the most significant benefits of his career by refueling his body with a lot of energy and an easy ladder to climb up on higher weight class and winning the title against a competitor who contained 9-inch height and 45 kg weight benefit on David Haye. But his amazing skills and high energy provided by the sirtfood diet provided him with the new world heavyweight title. It is enough to describe the benefits of the sirtfood diet.

Jodie Kidd

Jodie Kidd is a British celebrity and supermodel who started her modeling career in just 16 years of age. At that time, she was 6 feet and 1 inch tall, with just 48 kg of body weight. Her slender physique was very famous among girls, and it was also reported that some girls turned anorexic after following her beauty standards. She took eight months from her modeling career and started eating a more caloric diet, so; size 14 was achieved in dresses worn by Jodie Kidd in those eight months. She was slender, and her most significant issue was putting on some weight rather than losing it. So, it was much different than introduced by nearly all fat loss diets. She has to put some weight while keeping the total body fat percentage low and increasing the lean muscle mass. It is not less than a fat loss challenge, and physique like Jodie Kidd had, it was even more challenging to achieve that goal. She has made multiple transformations over the course of years. She is not only a supermodel but also a fast car racer and a television host. When asked from Jodie about her perfect shape and glowing skin, she said that all credits belong to the sirtfood diet. Interestingly, the sirtfood diet was thought of as a principle fat loss diet, but Jodie used this diet to put lean muscle mass on her making her more curvaceous and healthy-looking.

Jodie said that the sirtfood diet was a game-changer for her. She followed that regime and got the best shape of her life. It was hard to put weight on her lean body, but the sirtfood diet helped her to achieve her fitness goals. She mentioned that the sirtfood diet is the key behind her good looks. These statements in favor of the sirtfood diet made this diet even more popular among the fans of Jodie, and thousands of people started using this dieting regime.

James Haskell

James Haskell is a former professional rugby player who played for many years as a leading rugby star from the national rugby team of the UK. He was a fantastic rugby player in both under 16 and under 18 categories. James also played as a national rugby player from Wales and Ireland. He has one of the most successful careers in rugby. James Haskell is known for his incredible athletic energy and buffed physique. He has excellent lean muscle mass on his well-ripped body and a very low-fat percentage. James has maintained his physique for years keeping the right track on his diet and eating habits. His career of rugby is charming, and now he has a high motivation to compete as a pro-MMA fighter. He will compete in the heavyweight class in May 2020 and has firm hopes about a charming career in MMA as well. James Haskell has used the sirtfood diet to keep up his body according to the standards of the heavyweight class. His statement about the sirtfood diet is very famous as he claimed that the most excellent performances of his career in the 2015 rugby world cup were due to the sirtfood diet. He trained hard and smart by keeping the sirtfood diet on the table, and this leads to incredible energy levels in his body. This statement made the sirtfood diet extremely famous among his fans as well as among his competitors, and thousands of people have followed this diet plan to achieve the best in their lives.

Sir Ben Ainslie

Sir Ben Ainslie is the best sailor among the history of Great Britain. He is a British national who competed in many Olympic Games and won many titles to his names. He was a sailor when he was eight years old, and he competed internationally in Japan at the age of twelve. In 1196 he won the first Olympic gold medal in sailing. The unique capabilities of Sir Ben Ainslie are scarce, and Ben holds medals in five different categories of sailing sports. He is one of three athletes worldwide historically who achieved this rank. Moreover, Ben is the second-best Olympic sailor who holds four gold medals in sailing sports. He is a well-known athlete of British history and praised by millions of fans. The statements of Sir Ben Ainslie about the sirtfood diet are very supportive, and Ben mentioned the sirtfood diet as the vital force behind his successful career. He said that the sirtfood diet helped him achieving the best shape of his life and the best performances of his career because of the fantastic energy and focused mind. His performances in the British-American cup are the most golden memories of his career, and he claims that the sirtfood diet helped him achieve his goals in perfection.

Adele

Last but not least, Adele and the sirtfood diet is probably the most fantastic story of 2020 in context to physical transformations. Adele belongs to the UK, and she has won the best singer awards throughout her career. She is no doubt one of the loveliest voices in English pop history. She has amazing vocals and a very charming personality. Adele is one of those celebrities who have struggled a lot to achieve a lean physique, but it was never easy for her before the sirtfood diet. She was chubby and got plenty of extra pounds on her body. She was quite happy with her outlook, but she is also aware of the health risks associated with high body fat percentages. Adele has reportedly lost nearly 40 pounds of extra fat from her body within a few months of following the sirtfood diet. This diet plan was also popular among many other celebrities, but the transformation shown by Adele created an incredible hype of the sirtfood diet. She now has the best shape of her life and a fantastic body, which is much leaner and healthier than before. Adele is very vocal about the health benefits of the sirtfood diet, and because of her vast transformation, the sirtfood diet is known as "The Adele Diet".

So, these statements are enough to show the benefits associated with the sirtfood diet, and when used properly, the sirtfood diet can be a great precursor behind the success of your life-changing achievements.

Conclusion

In spite of the fact that the eating regimen is frequently hailed as simple to follow on account of the reality, it incorporates red wine and dull chocolate, it's genuinely severe in its rules. The sirtfood plan depends on health food nuts confining their calorie admission just as eating a particular rundown of nourishments that are said to help the digestion.

An eating routine that stresses dim chocolate, red wine, kale, berries, and espresso? It either seems like the most ideal street to health and weight reduction, or unrealistic. Be that as it may, pause, it shows signs of improvement: According to the makers of the Sirtfood Diet, these and other alleged "sirtfoods" are indicated to enact the systems constrained by your body's characteristic "thin qualities" to assist you with consuming fat and get fit.

Bragging rundown delicious nourishment, you likely as of now love, and supported by reports that Adele utilized it to shed pounds in the wake of having an infant, the Sirtfood Diet sounds justifiably engaging.

In any case, not to demolish your chocolate-and-red-wine high here, yet the science doesn't really bolster the eating regimen's greatest cases. Which isn't to state that eating sirtfoods is an impractical notion... in any case, similarly as with all eating regimens that sound unrealistic, you should take a gander at this one with the genuine investigation. This is what you have to think about what sirtfoods can and can't accomplish for you.

Created by U.K. nourishment experts Aidan Goggin's and Glen Matten, the Sirtfood Diet accentuates plant-based food sources that are known "certain activators." Basically, when you nosh on the arrangement's key fixings, you invigorate the proteins encoded for by the SIRT1 quality, which Goggin's and Matten have named "the thin quality."

SIRT1 and certain proteins are accepted to assume a job in maturing and life span, which might be identified with the defensive impacts of calorie limitation. The case behind the Sirtfood Diet is that sure nourishments can actuate these sort-intervened pathways sans the limitation, and in this way "switch on your muscle to fat ratio's consuming forces, supercharge weight reduction, and help fight off malady."

Alongside red wine, dull chocolate, berries, espresso, and kale, certain-advancing nourishments incorporate matcha green tea, additional virgin olive oil, pecans, parsley, red onions, soy, and turmeric (a.k.a. incredible flavors and go-to solid treats).

There's some science behind the cases of sirtfoods' advantages, yet it's exceptionally constrained and rather dubious. The science on the shirt outskirts is still overly new. There are examines investigating the SIRT1 quality's job in maturing and life span, in maturing related weight increase and maturing related malady, and in shielding the heart from irritation brought about by a high-fat eating routine. However, the exploration is constrained to work done in test tubes and on mice, which is not adequate proof to state that certain-boosting nourishments can have weight reduction or hostile to maturing abilities in a real human body.

Brooke Alpert, R.D., creator of The Sugar Detox, says there's an exploration to recommend that the weight-control advantages of sirtfoods may come to a limited extent from the polyphenol-cancer prevention agent resveratrol, frequently advertised as a component in red wine. "All things considered, it is difficult to devour enough red wine to get benefits," she says, taking note of that she does as often as possible recommend resveratrol enhancements to her customers.

Furthermore, some nourishment specialists aren't psyched about the manner in which the Sirtfood Diet plan works.

As per top dietitians who've surveyed the arrangement, the Sirtfood Diet is feeling the loss of some significant components for a solid, adjusted routine. Goggin's and Matten's eating routine arrangement includes three stages: a couple of days at 1,000 calories for each day, comprised of one sirtfood-overwhelming feast and green squeezes; a couple of long stretches of two sirtfood suppers and two squeezes every day, for an aggregate of 1,500 calories; and a fourteen-day support period of thirty dinners and juices. The decision? Sirtfoods are incredible to have in your eating routine, however, they shouldn't be all you have.

There's positively no explanation you can't include some sirtfoods into your eating plan, says Alpert. "I think there are some truly fascinating things here, similar to the red wine, dim chocolate, matcha—I love these things," she says. "I love mentioning to individuals what to concentrate on rather than what to nix from their eating routine." If it tastes liberal and it's solid in little amounts, why not?

Be that as it may, all the nourishment specialists propose balancing the eating regimen with some lean protein and sound fats, for example, progressively nuts and seeds, avocado, and greasy fish like salmon. Stir up your plate of mixed greens game, as well, with more kinds of veggies, spinach, and romaine lettuce notwithstanding the kale and red onions. Primary concern? The majority of the sirtfoods are an ok to eat and solid for you, however, simply do not depend on the eating routine to actuate any "thin quality" presently.

"We don't yet have the proof that specific nourishments actuate this more than others – or to which specific tissues they'd be gainful," says. "Regardless of whether sirtfoods do help to weight loss, the sheer amount we'd have to eat might be unmanageable." He focuses on resveratrol, the polyphenol in red wine and the most notable of all sirtuin activators.

Resveratrol shot to popularity in 2003 when a research facility of researchers run by David Sinclair found that this compound, found most normally in the skins of red grapes, copied the impacts of calorie limitation and actuated sirtuins that drawn-out the life of cells. Subsequently, the 'red wine encourages you to live more' way of thinking that is become progressively mainstream bandied about at the bar.

Be that as it may, Hirschey brings up, 'most of the studies have been done utilizing test frameworks in the lab, generally on mice or natural product flies, or legitimately into cells. To get resveratrol's enemy of maturing impacts from red wine, you'd need to drink up to 40 liters every day.' Which makes you wonder how much kale you'd pack so as to get thinner.

The nutraceutical business is as of now one stage ahead, with resveratrol supplements effectively accessible. Be watchful, in any case, of simply popping some sirt-enacting pills or binding your smoothies with resveratrol powder, as one examination from the University of Copenhagen has demonstrated that expanded supplementation of the cancer prevention agent neutralized the great impacts of the activity.

Actually, you don't need to, particularly not to begin. Currently, we are adapted to be snappy and proficient, and to be brisk, we have been acquainted with inexpensive food and handled nourishment.

I think what many individuals foul up as do I (during the time spent fixing my diet) is to think about the nourishment being removed, so obviously with that sort of reasoning, it turns out to be almost difficult to go for a superfood/raw food diet. Be that as it may, if we have a go at including the superfood/raw food into our current diet, things like crude vegetables, sprouts, natural products, and juices, you won't experience considerable difficulties exchanging. In the wake of adding these natural products to your diet, you may not be as eager and when you're not ravenous, you won't surrender to purchasing inexpensive food and prepared nourishment.

Since you will have more opportunity to consider your buys and you have gotten increasingly acclimated with eating more advantageous. If you need that steak or even a McDonald's cheeseburger, you can get yourself it, and it will taste so much better... or on the other hand, you might be fortunate to the point that you won't need it by any stretch of the imagination. When you begin eating Superfoods, however, you will begin to see how great you feel and the amount more vitality you have, that cheeseburger just won't look as great to you any longer.

During the time spent changing your diet and after changing you would like no doubt, however, that you're getting enough of the correct sorts of sustenance. Eating Superfoods/crude nourishments isn't simply enough you have to do some exploration on the most proficient method to add your fundamental proteins to your new diet. Recall before you got your protein through your meat yet now you need to get it through your vegetables and crude nourishment, so you have to recognize what to eat and what blends you have to eat to get enough proteins.

One approach to do this is to present another vegetable or crude dish each week. If you are to purchase another vegetable every week and become acclimated to the taste by utilizing it in your feast the entire week. By doing this you will adjust to the new tastes and surfaces and you will begin feeling more regrettable and more terrible for each time you go for inexpensive food or handled nourishment.

Did you enjoy this book?

If you enjoyed this book, it would be awesome if you could leave a quick review on Amazon. Your feedback is much appreciated and I would love to hear from you.

<u>Leave a Review on Amazon</u>

Thanks so much!!

More books by Geena Moore:

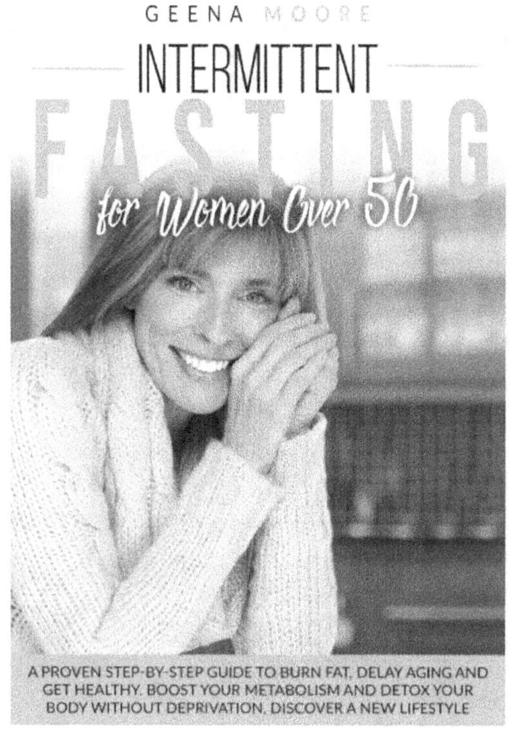

Intermittent Fasting for Women Over 50: A Proven Step-By-Step Guide to Burn Fat, Delay Aging and Get Healthy. Boost Your Metabolism and Detox Your Body without Deprivation, Discover a New Lifestyle. (Link)

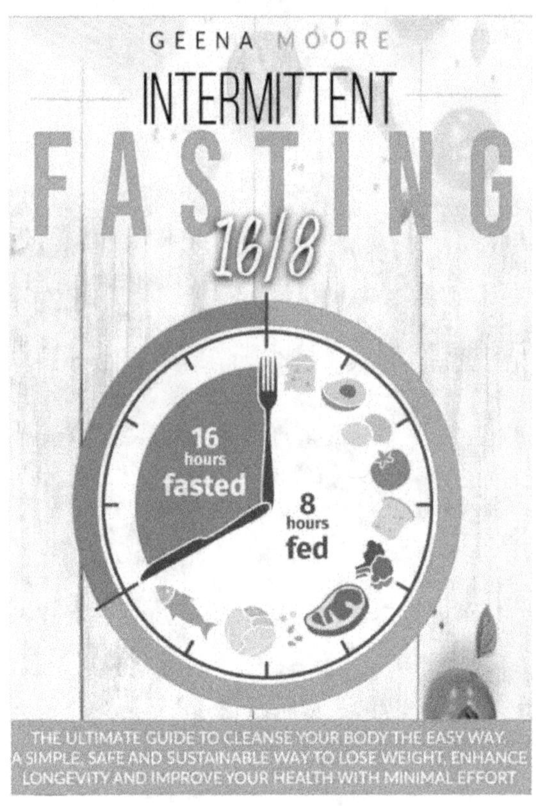

Intermittent Fasting 16/8: The Ultimate Guide To Cleanse Your Body The Easy Way. A Simple, Safe and Sustainable Way to Lose Weight, Enhance Longevity and Improve Your Health with Minimal Effort. (Link)